Type 1 and Type 2 Diabetes

Type 1 and Type 2 Diabetes

Editor: Solomon Fleming

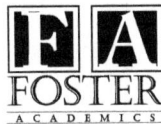

FA
FOSTER
ACADEMICS

www.fosteracademics.com

www.fosteracademics.com

F A
FOSTER
A C A D E M I C S

Cataloging-in-Publication Data

Type 1 and type 2 diabetes / edited by Solomon Fleming.
    p. cm.
Includes bibliographical references and index.
ISBN 978-1-63242-649-9
1. Diabetes. 2. Non-insulin-dependent diabetes. I. Fleming, Solomon.
RC660 .T97 2019
6164--dc23

Foster Academics,
118-35 Queens Blvd., Suite 400,
Forest Hills, NY 11375, USA

ISBN 978-1-63242-649-9 (Hardback)

Contents

Preface

It is often said that books are a boon to mankind. They document every progress and pass on the knowledge from one generation to the other. They play a crucial role in our lives. Thus I was both excited and nervous while editing this book. I was pleased by the thought of being able to make a mark but I was also nervous to do it right because the future of students depends upon it. Hence, I took a few months to research further into the discipline, revise my knowledge and also explore some more aspects. Post this process, I begun with the editing of this book.

Diabetes mellitus Type 1 or Type 1 diabetes is a type of diabetes mellitus, which is caused by little or no production of insulin by the pancreas. This leads to high blood sugar levels in the body. Such a high blood sugar level is typically an autoimmune response involving a loss of insulin-producing beta cells in the pancreas. Diabetes mellitus Type 2 or Type 2 diabetes is a metabolic disorder caused due to insulin resistance, high sugar levels in blood and comparatively low insulin production. It is the most common form of diabetes and makes up nearly 90% of all cases of diabetes. Genetics and lifestyle are the major contributing factors for the incidence of Type 1 and Type 2 diabetes. Symptoms for both these disorders are similar. These include weight loss, frequent urination, increased thirst and hunger, etc. This book provides comprehensive insights into Type 1 and Type 2 diabetes. It discusses the fundamentals as well as modern approaches in the management of these disorders. For all those who are interested in endocrinology and metabolism, this book can prove to be an essential guide.

I thank my publisher with all my heart for considering me worthy of this unparalleled opportunity and for showing unwavering faith in my skills. I would also like to thank the editorial team who worked closely with me at every step and contributed immensely towards the successful completion of this book. Last but not the least, I wish to thank my friends and colleagues for their support.

Editor

Management of Diabetic Retinopathy and Other Ocular Complications in Type 1 Diabetes

Efraim Berco, Daniel Rappoport, Ayala Pollack, Guy Kleinmann and Yoel Greenwald

Abstract

Type 1 diabetes can reduce vision by affecting various parts of the eye. Proactive, interdisciplinary coordination of treatment and timely referrals can aid in the minimization of visually threatening complications, significantly enhancing patient quality of life. The main causes of visual impairment in diabetes are proliferative diabetic retinopathy and macular edema. Until recently, the mainstay of treatment for both conditions was retinal laser, which prevented significant vision loss but was much less effective at improving vision, especially in macular edema. Over the past decade, exciting new advances in treating diabetic eye disease, namely intraocular steroid and antivascular endothelial growth factor injections, have greatly improved the visual prognosis for the majority of patients with diabetic eye disease.

Keywords: Diabetic retinopathy, Macular edema, Laser, Intraocular injection, Cataract

1. Introduction

Type 1 diabetes is a complex metabolic disease that involves multiple organ systems which can cause severe visual impairment. Almost all ocular structures may be afflicted in diabetes including: the extraocular muscles, the intraocular lens, the optic nerve, and the retina.

Diabetes is the leading cause of blindness between the ages of 20 and 74 in many developed countries. Individuals with diabetes are 25 times more likely to become legally blind than individuals without diabetes. The aspect of diabetic eye disease most responsible for vision loss is diabetic retinopathy, which accounts for ¼ of blind registrations in the Western world [1,2]. There are two main pathways by which diabetic retinopathy affects vision; fluid accumulation in the center of vision, or macular edema, and the formation of pathological retinal vessels also known as proliferative diabetic retinopathy.

Prevention of severe visual impairment in type 1 diabetes includes: optimal glycemic control, the treatment of ancillary risk factors such as hypertension, and regular screening for early diagnosis and treatment of ocular complications.

In the following chapter, we will describe how diabetes affects different ocular structures and discuss the treatment options available today to combat these complications.

2. Extraocular muscles

Patients with diabetes may present with a sudden onset of diplopia (double vision). This is usually caused by a paresis of one of the extraocular muscles due to microvascular damage to the third, fourth, or the sixth cranial nerves [3,4].

When the extraocular muscle deficit is due to microvascular complications of diabetes the prognosis is good. Recovery of ocular motor function generally begins within three months of onset and recovery is usually complete. Although the diplopia can be debilitating, due to the generally limited course of these complaints, patients can usually be effectively managed conservatively with eye patching. When diplopia is from large divergence of the visual axes, patching one eye is the only practical short-term solution. When the deviation is smaller, the diplopia often can be resolved by using glasses with a horizontal or vertical prism or both. Surgery is rarely indicated.

If patients do not recover from a cranial nerve palsy within 6-12 months, eye muscle surgery to treat persistent and stable angle diplopia should be considered. These patients should consult with a neuro-ophthalmologist for continuing care.

3. Intraocular lens: Cataract

Cataract is a common cause of visual impairment in patients with diabetes. The Framingham study [5] revealed a three- to four fold increased prevalence of cataract in diabetic patients under the age of 65, and up to a twofold increased prevalence in patients above 65. Duration of diabetes and quality of glycemic control are the major risk factors for early cataract development [5].

Recurrent high levels of glucose in the lens lead to the glycolation of lens proteins from increased nonenzymatic glycation and oxidative stress to the lens [6]. This causes diabetic patients to develop age-related lens changes similar to nondiabetic age-related cataracts, except that they tend to occur at a younger age [7]. Several studies have analyzed the effect of vitamin and antioxidant supplements, such as vitamin C, E, and beta carotene and zinc, on preventing or slowing progression of age-related cataracts in diabetes without showing any statistically significant benefit with their use [6].

Early cataracts may cause mild visual impairment that can be managed reasonably with spectacle correction. Cataract surgery is indicated when visual function is significantly impaired by the cataract or if the cataract obscures the view of the retina and makes the diagnosis and treatment of diabetic retinopathy difficult.

Cataract surgery is safe in diabetic patients and there is a 95% success rate in terms of improved visual acuity [6]. Good glycemic control, fluid and electrolyte balance should be maintained perioperatively and the patient's treating physician and anesthesiologist should be involved in the process. It is recommended that the surgery be scheduled in the morning to minimize changes in the patient's usual schedule [8].

Some controversy exists regarding a potential association between cataract surgery and a subsequent worsening of diabetic retinopathy. Patients should be made aware of this risk preoperatively. Cataract surgery and its effect on diabetic retinopathy will be discussed in more detail in section 7.3.2.

4. Cornea

Corneal disorders secondary to diabetes (diabetic keratopathy) are increasingly recognized as a cause of ocular morbidity associated with diabetes. Patients with diabetes have structural changes of the corneal basement membrane that contributes to defects in the adhesion of corneal epithelial cells to the deeper stromal tissue [9]. This increases the risk of recurrent corneal erosions. In addition, accumulation of sorbitol in the cornea during periods of hyperglycemia leads to hypoesthesia (a loss of corneal sensation). Both hypoesthesia and epithelial adhesion dysfunction occur more frequently with increased severity and duration of diabetes. In patients with more long-standing or advanced diabetes, any corneal epithelial injury, either from trauma, during ocular surgery or from routine contact lens use, may result in prolonged healing times. This increases the risk of severe complications such as bacterial infiltration and ulceration.

Treatment of diabetic keratopathy is multifaceted, including artificial tears for mild cases, and the use of topical antibiotics, a bandage contact lens, eye patching, or closure for more severe cases.

5. Iris

Rubeosis iridis, neovascularization of the iris, is a serious complication of diabetes which occurs in patients with severe diabetic retinopathy [3]. Severe retinal ischemia stimulates the formation of numerous intertwining blood vessels on the anterior surface of the iris. These vessels can block aqueous outflow from the anterior chamber, leading to a sharp and persistent rise in intraocular pressure. This complication is known as neovascular glaucoma. This type of glaucoma is hard to treat and is often associated with pain from very high ocular pressure.

Topical medical therapy used commonly in other forms of glaucoma is less effective. Treatment should include aggressive control of the underlying diabetic retinopathy. The treatment of diabetic retinopathy will be discussed in more detail in section 7.

6. Retina – Diabetic retinopathy

Damage to the retinal capillaries, known as diabetic retinopathy, is the hallmark of diabetic eye disease. This condition is the major cause of blindness and visual disability in patients with type 1 diabetes.

There are two main pathways by which diabetic retinopathy can reduce vision: macular edema and proliferative retinopathy. These conditions can appear concomitantly or separately with the treatment protocol tailored to the relative severity each condition.

Macular edema develops when damaged retina vessels leak fluid and protein. These deposits collect on or under the macula of the eye where central vision is processed. This causes the macula to thicken and swell and may distort central vision.

Proliferative retinopathy occurs when diffuse injury to retinal vessels severely impairs retinal oxygenation. The hypoxia induces the release of proteins which stimulate the growth (or proliferation) of new, fragile retinal vessels. These new vessels have a propensity to bleed, which severely reduces vision.

In the following sections, we will discuss how retinopathy and macular edema develop and the various treatment options available to patients today, with a focus on exciting recent developments.

6.1. Epidemiology

Diabetic retinopathy is one of the most frequent causes of preventable blindness in working aged adults (20-74 years) [1,10]. In the USA, an estimated 86% of patients with type 1 diabetes have some degree of diabetic retinopathy. Data from the Wisconsin Epidemiologic Study of Diabetic Retinopathy (WESDR) showed that within 5 years of diagnosis of type 1 diabetes, 14% of patients developed retinopathy, with the incidence rising to 74% by 10 years [11,12]. In people with retinopathy at the WESDR baseline examination, 64% had their retinopathy worsen, 17% progressed to proliferative diabetic retinopathy (PDR), and about 20% developed diabetic macular edema during 10 years of follow-up.

The WESDR data in type 1 diabetics showed that 25 years after diagnosis, 97% of patients developed retinopathy, 43% progressed to PDR, 29% developed diabetic macular edema, and 3.6% of patients younger than 30 at diagnosis were legally blind [11]. The WESDR results also showed a reduction in the yearly incidence and progression of diabetic retinopathy during the past 15 years [12]. This may be signaling an improved ocular prognosis for diabetics today, possibly due to recent advances in glycemic control, ophthalmic treatment, and patient education.

The course of diabetic retinal disease in children with type 1 diabetes is fairly benign. Severe vision-reducing complications are uncommon in children before puberty [13].

6.2. Risk factors

There are several risk factors which influence the development and progression of diabetic retinopathy. The following list contains most of the important risk factors known today.

Modifiable risk factors:

1. **Hyperglycemia**: Good glycemic control has been shown to significantly prevent the development and progression of diabetic retinopathy. Every 1% decrease in hemoglobin A_{1C} leads to a 40% reduction in the risk of developing retinopathy, a 25% reduction in the risk of progression to vision-threatening retinopathy, and a 15% reduction in the risk of blindness [1,14,15].

2. **Hypertension**: Good blood pressure control is important in reducing the risk of retinopathy. Every 10 mmHg reduction in systolic blood pressure leads to a reduction of 35% in the risk of retinopathy progression and a reduction of 50% in the risk of visual loss [1].

3. **Obesity**: Obesity (BMI>30 kg/m(2)) is an important risk factor for diabetic retinopathy progression in type 1 diabetes, independent of HbA1c levels [16].

4. **Smoking**: There is some evidence that smoking may be a risk factor in progression of retinopathy in type 1 diabetes [17].

Nonmodifiable risk factors:

1. **Diabetes duration**: The longer the duration of diabetes, the higher the risk of developing diabetic retinopathy and of having a severe manifestation of this disease [1].

2. **Genetic factors**: The Diabetes Control and Complications Trial [18] showed a heritable tendency for developing diabetic retinopathy, regardless of other risk factors. The abnormal development of new blood vessels is regulated by protein called vascular endothelial growth factor A (VEGF –A). Variation in the sequence of this gene is associated with the development of severe diabetic retinopathy [19].

3. **Ethnicity**: Diabetic retinopathy in America is more prevalent among African Americans, Hispanic and south Asian groups than in Caucasians with otherwise similar risk profiles [1].

4. **Gender**: there is an observed gender dimorphism with younger females being at greater risk for diabetic retinopathy early in the course of diabetes [20] and males demonstrating greater risk later in life [21].

Other risk factors:

Pregnancy: Pregnancy is associated with worsening of diabetic retinopathy [22]. All pregnant women need to be closely monitored throughout pregnancy. Pregnancy in type 1 diabetes is discussed in further detail in section 7.3.1.

6.3. Pathophysiology

Diabetic retinopathy develops when hyperglycemia and other causal risk factors trigger a cascade of biochemical changes which damage retinal blood vessels. Hyperglycemia increases sorbitol levels via the action of aldose reductase increasing oxidative stress by reducing intracellular levels of reduced glutathione, an important antioxidant [23]. Intracellular hyperglycemia also increases synthesis of diacylglycerol, an activating cofactor for protein kinase C (PKC). Activated PKC decreases the production of anti-artherosclerotic factors and increases production of pro-arthogenic factors, pro-adhesive and pro-inflammatory factors [23]. As well, intracellular hyperglycemia leads to a rise in intracellular N-acetylglucosamine levels. This by-product reacts with serine and threonine residues in transcription factors, resulting in pathologic changes in gene expression [23]. The final by-product of these pathological processes is increased inflammation and increased oxidative stress, which causes endothelial cell dysfunction in retinal blood vessels.

Endothelial cell dysfunction induces retinal arteriolar dilatation, which increases capillary bed pressure. This results in microaneurysm formation, vessel leakage, and rupture [1]. Vascular permeability is also increased from loss of pericytes and increased endothelial proliferation in retinal capillaries. The breakdown of the blood–retinal barrier allows fluid to accumulate in the deep retinal layers where it damages photoreceptors and other neural tissues. This is the mechanism by which macular edema reduces visual acuity.

In some capillaries there is endothelial cell apoptosis. Vessels become acellular, leading to vascular occlusion and nonperfusion of local retinal tissue [23]. The resultant retinal ischemia promotes the release of inflammatory growth factors, such as vascular endothelial growth factor, growth-hormone-insulin growth factor, and erythropoietin [1]. These factors influence neovascularization, the growth of new capillaries, which are generally ineffective in improving tissue oxygenation as they often grow up toward the vitreous cavity.

6.4. Clinical features and classification

Diabetic retinopathy is classified as nonproliferative diabetic retinopathy (NPDR) when the vascular changes are limited to the retinal surface. It is classified as proliferative diabetic retinopathy (PDR) in the more advanced stage when new blood vessels form, which grow from the retinal surface up toward the vitreous cavity.

Diabetic macular edema occurs when leaky capillary beds allow fluid to accumulate in the part of the retina responsible for central vision. This complication can occur in patients with any level of underlying retinopathy from mild NPDR to severe PDR. Visual impairment is usually related to the state of macular disease and the consequences of neovascularization such as vitreous hemorrhage and retinal detachment. As such, the level of retinopathy does not always correlate with visual function, and severe diabetic retinopathy can be present initially without significant visual loss.

6.5. Diabetic macular edema

Diabetic macular edema (DME) is the complication of retinopathy responsible for most of the moderate visual loss in retinopathy patients. The loss of vision is often very mild at first, but without effective treatment it can progress and patients can lose the ability to perform activities of daily living such as reading and driving. Diabetic macular edema is assessed separately from the stage of retinopathy (NPDR/PDR) and it can manifest along a different and independent course.

The edema evolves when damage to the macular capillary bed causes increased retinal vascular permeability and fluid accumulation in the macula. Clinical examination can reveal rings of hard exudates (lipid-filled macrophages) that delineate the area of focal leakage.

Optical Coherence Tomography (OCT) is a useful ancillary imaging technique in DME. Recent technological advances in OCT technology have provided physicians with high-resolution images of the retina in cross-sectional slices. Aside from demonstrating areas of retinal thickening and intraretinal fluid, OCT obtains quantitative measurements of central retinal thickness. Serial OCT examinations are often used as a noninvasive and accurate method analyzing treatment response in DME patients [1].

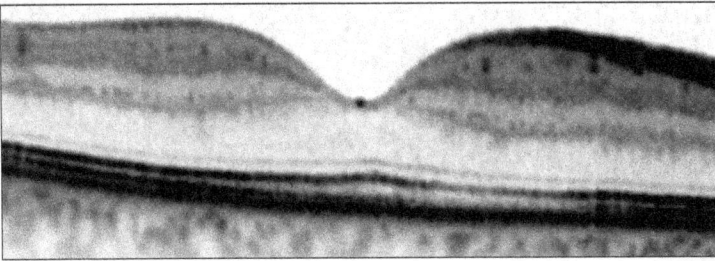

Figure 1. Normal OCT of the macular region.

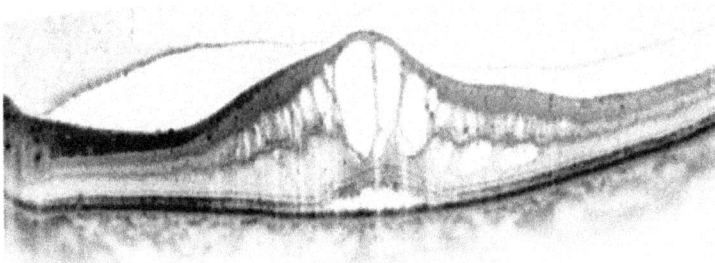

Figure 2. Macular edema: The OCT demonstrates the disruption of the normal macular anatomy due to macular edema.

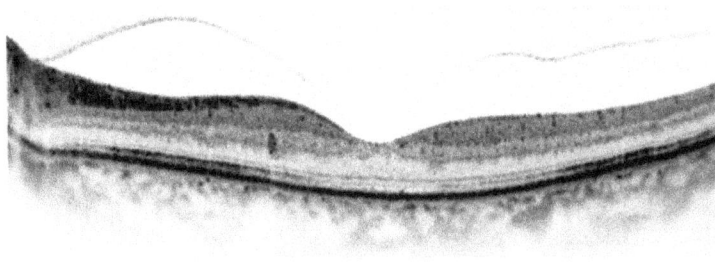

Figure 3. Posttreatment OCT: The same patient as in Figure 2 after treatment with intravitreal injections. The edema has been reabsorbed.

6.5.1. Nonproliferative Diabetic Retinopathy (NPDR)

In NPDR, the retinal microvascular changes do not extend beyond the surface of the retina. Clinical findings include microaneurysms (saccular enlargements of weakened capillaries), intraretinal hemorrhages, hard exudates (lipid-filled macrophages), cotton wool spots (nerve fiber layer infarcts), venous dilatations, and intraretinal microvascular abnormalities (dilated preexisting capillaries) [1,10].

NPDR is classified as mild, moderate, or severe, reflecting the risk of progression to PDR (Table 1) as determined by the Early Treatment in Diabetic Retinopathy Study [24].

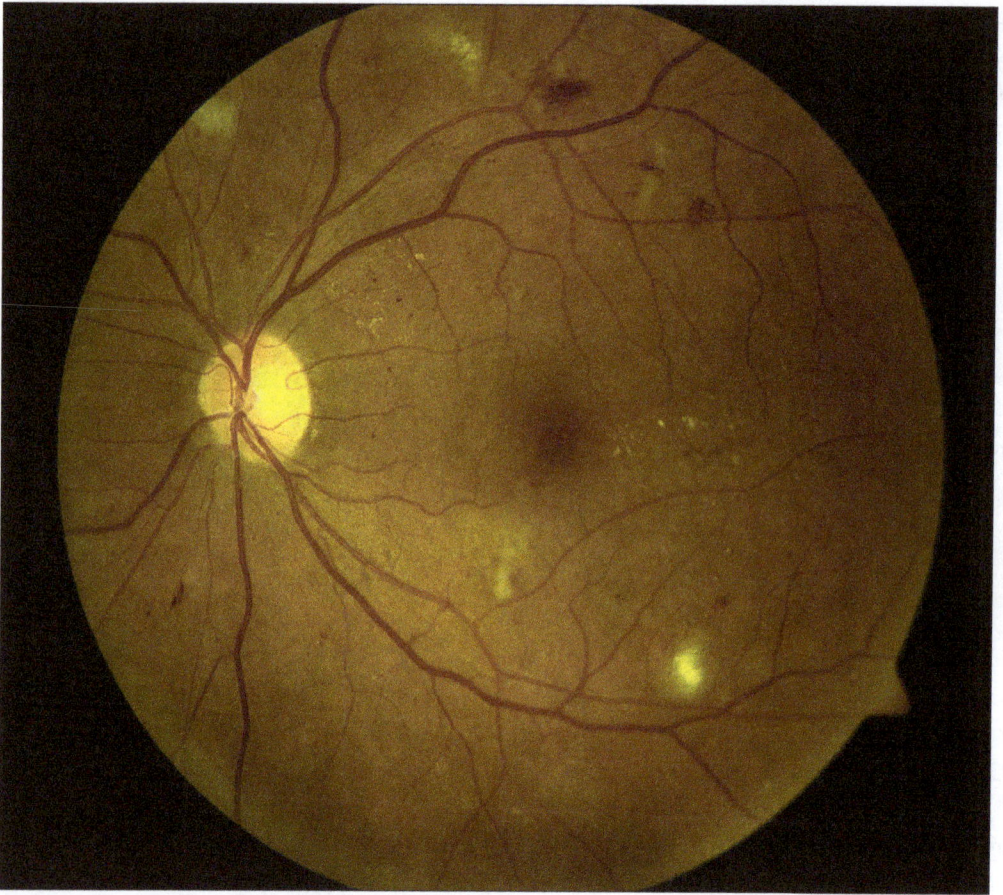

Figure 4. Nonproliferative diabetic retinopathy: Scattered hemorrhages ("dot and blot" shaped) can be seen throughout the retina.

6.5.2. Proliferative Diabetic Retinopathy (PDR)

Diabetic retinopathy advances to the proliferative stage when new vessels (neovascularizations) are formed which grow up from the retinal surface toward the vitreous cavity. The growth of these vessels is potentiated by the progression of diabetic retinal microvascular disease, causing severe retinal ischemia. This induces the release of proangiogenic factors which promote the growth of these pathological vessels. Neovascularizations can be identified clinically as a jumble of disorganized, fine vessels emanating from the organized retinal vessel architecture. Angiography is also very effective at identifying neovascular lesions as the new vessels are porous and leak fluorescent dye into the vitreous cavity.

The new vessels in PDR evolve in three stages. Initially, the fine new vessels grow with minimal fibrous tissue. Then the new vessels increase in gauge and length with an increased fibrous component. Finally, the vessels regress and the residual fibrovascular tissue along the posterior surface of the vitreous body contracts.

Retinal neovascularizations (NV) are divided into two subtypes based on their relative risk of causing severe visual loss as demonstrated by the Diabetic Retinopathy Study (DRS). Vascular proliferations on or near the optic disc are termed NV-disc (NVD) and proliferations elsewhere are termed NV-elsewhere (NVE). The presence of NVD carries the higher risk of severe visual loss and requires more urgent treatment [25,26].

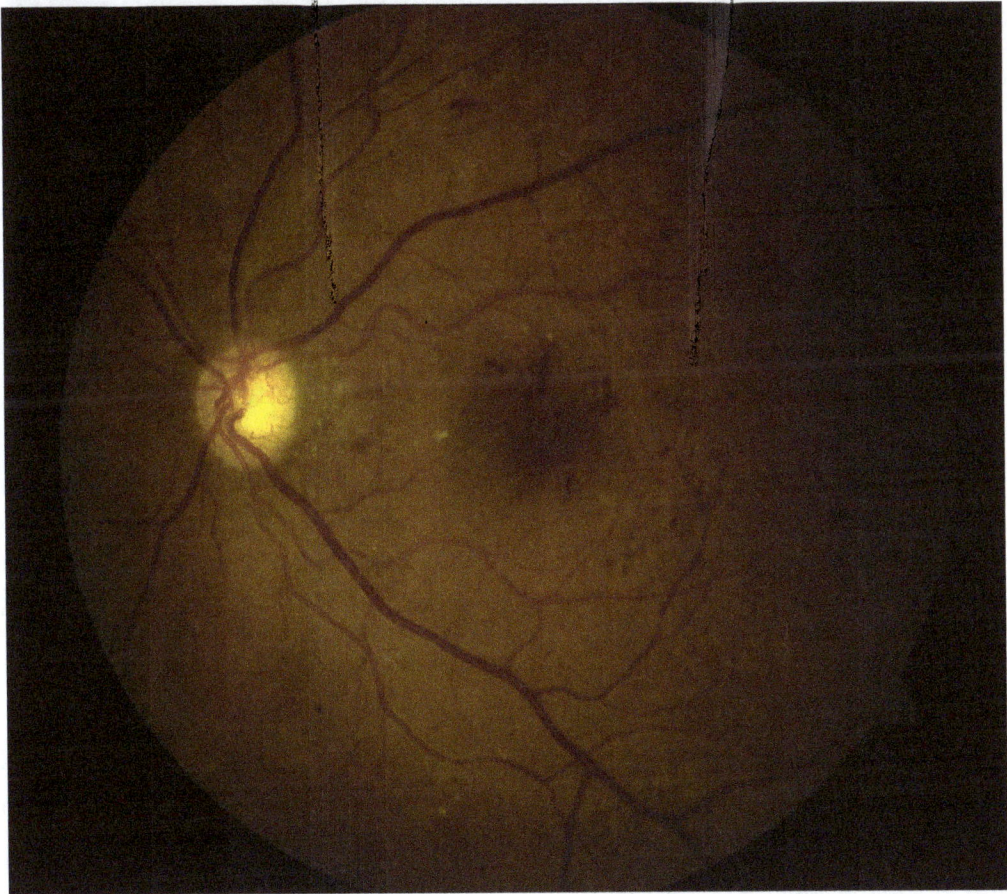

Figure 5. Neovascularization on the optic disc (NVD): The growth of fine new blood vessels can be seen on the optic disc. Urgent treatment is indicated to reduce the risk of vitreous hemorrhage.

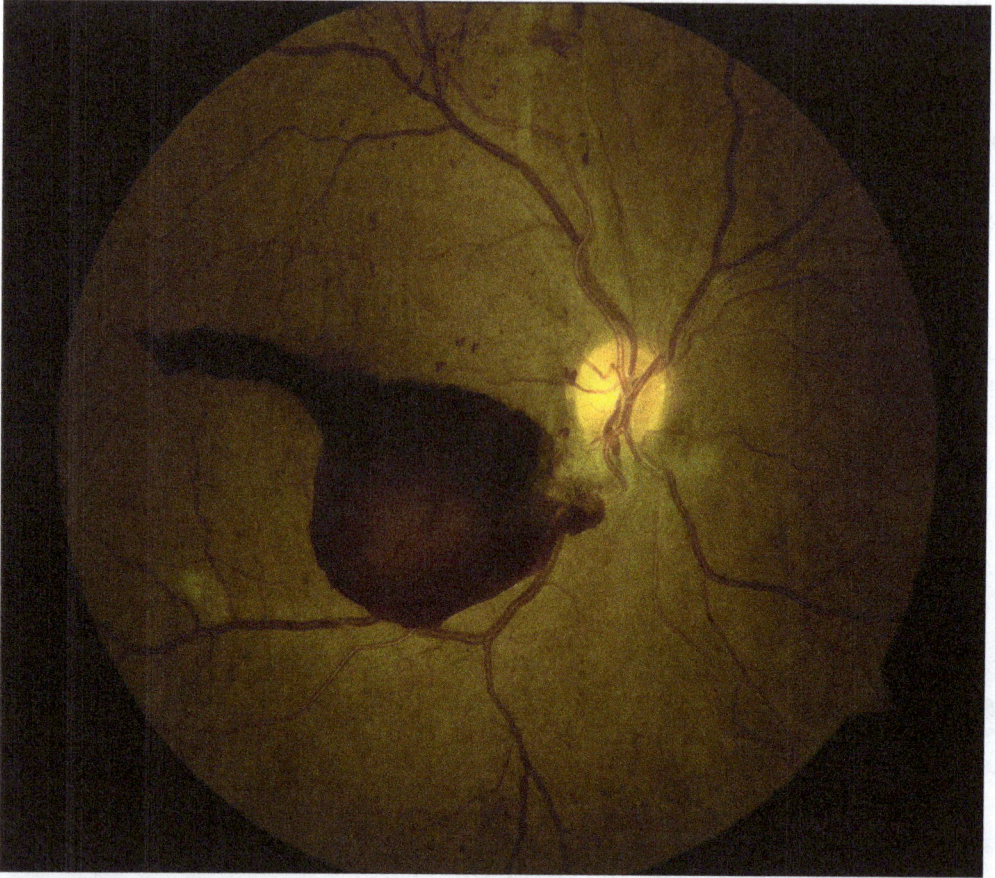

Figure 6. Vitreous hemorrhage with a neovascularization of the optic disc (NVD): The fragile blood vessels of the NVD have ruptured and a vitreous hemorrhage has collected, partially obscuring the macula and severely limiting vision.

PDR is graded from early to high risk according to the extent of the neovascular proliferations. The DRS [25,26] defined high-risk PDR as the presence of either: NVD with a vitreous hemorrhage, NVD larger than a quarter disc area without vitreous hemorrhage, or NVE larger than half disc area with vitreous hemorrhage. Without treatment, patients with early PDR have 50% risk of developing high-risk PDR in 1 year and those with high-risk PDR have a 25% risk of severe visual loss within 2 years. Treatment of PDR involving extensive peripheral laser ablation of the retina is discussed section 7.2.3.

The most common complication of PDR is vitreous hemorrhage caused by bleeding from the pathological neovascular vessels. Retinal detachments can also occur from the contraction of the neovascular tissue connecting the retinal surface to the vitreous.

Visual acuity in the absence of macular disease is often very good in PDR until a complication occurs; most commonly vitreous hemorrhage. This sudden transition from good vision to near blindness is often traumatic for patients who were unaware of the severity of their diabetic eye disease.

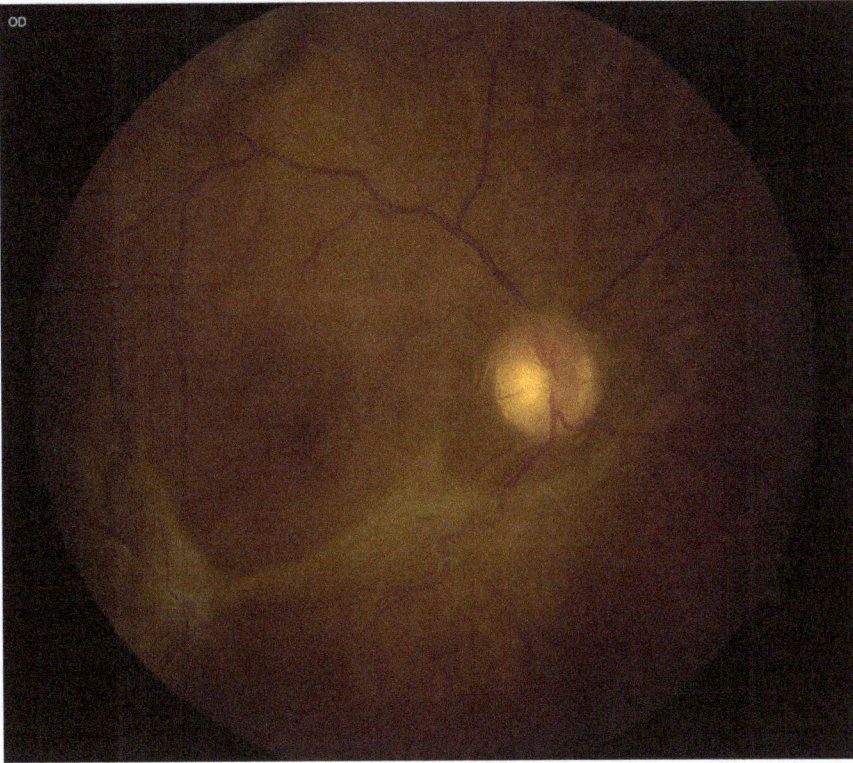

Figure 7. Traction Retinal Detachment: The neovascular tissue emanating from the optic disc and elsewhere has regressed leaving behind white fibrous tissue. This tissue has contracted and is distorting the retina in the macular region.

	Clinical Features	Progression Risk
Mild NPDR	Few microaneurysms	5% progress to PDR within 1 year
Moderate NPDR	Microaneurysms and other microvascular lesions	12-16% progress to PDR within 1 year
Severe NPDR (Meets 1 of 3 criteria)	• Extensive intraretinal hemorrhages and microaneurysms in all four quadrants • Venous beading in two or more quadrants • One IRMA	52% progress to PDR within 1 year 15% progress to high risk PDR within 1 year
Very severe NPDR	Any two of the features of severe NPDR	75% progress to PDR within 1 year 45% progress to high risk PDR within 1 year
Early PDR		50% risk of developing high risk PDR in 1 year
High risk PDR		25% risk of severe visual loss within 2 years

Table 1. Clinical classification of nonproliferative and proliferative diabetic retinopathy

7. Treatment of diabetic retinopathy

The main goal of treatment of diabetic retinopathy is to prevent complications that can lead to vision loss. Treatment should include both ocular therapy and systemic medical intervention.

7.1. Medical treatment

Hyperglycemia, hypertension, and hyperlipidemia are known risk factors for the development and progression of diabetic retinopathy. Treating and controlling these factors is crucial to preventing and limiting disease progression.

The Diabetes Control and Complications Trial [14] showed that intensive glycemic control reduced both the risk of developing retinopathy and the rate of progression of existing retinopathy. Intensive glycemic control reduced the risk for progression to severe NPDR and PDR, and the incidence of diabetic macular edema. Every percent reduction in hemoglobin A_{1C} lowers the risk of retinopathy development by 30-40%.

Antihypertensive treatment with ACE (angiotensin-converting enzyme) inhibitors can slow progression of diabetic nephropathy. The EUCLID study [27] investigated the effect of Lisinopril on progression of retinopathy in normotensive type 1 diabetics. They found that Lisinopril can decrease retinopathy progression in nonhypertensive patients who have type 1 diabetes with little or no nephropathy, although the mechanism is unclear. Unfortunately, other studies investigating the effect of ACE inhibitors on the progression of DR in type 1 diabetics have shown no significant benefits.

7.2. Ocular therapy

Ocular therapy in diabetic retinopathy includes panretinal or focal laser photocoagulation, intravitreal injections of either steroids or inhibitors of Vascular Endothelial Growth Factor (VEGF), surgery, or a combination of the aforementioned treatments. The suitable treatment regimen must be tailored individually for each patient and is based on clinical status of the patient (ocular and systemic), previous treatments, and data from the several reported and ongoing studies.

7.2.1. Diabetic macular edema treatment

Treatment options for diabetic macular edema (DME) include focal laser photocoagulation, intravitreal injections of either steroids or anti-VEGF compounds, and surgery.

7.2.1.1. Focal laser treatment

Until recently, the mainstay of DME treatment was macular laser photocoagulation. Treatment criteria are based on the ETDRS recommendations [24], which showed that eyes with macular edema involving or adjacent to the central macula, defined as clinically significant macular edema (CSME), benefited from macular laser treatment. Laser treatment reduced the risk of moderate visual loss (loss of three lines of vision) by 50% over 2 years compared with no treatment [24].

Macular laser treatment for CSME involves the application of discrete laser burns to areas of leakage in the macula. The treatment is not painful and can be repeated up to every 4 months.

Side effects of macular laser photocoagulation include: visual field loss, choroidal neovascularization, subretinal fibrosis, and inadvertent foveolar burns [10].

Modified photocoagulation techniques have been developed in response to these potential complications. The target of macular laser treatment for CSME is retinal pigment epithelium (RPE). Ideally, the laser energy would be absorbed only by the RPE and not spread to the surrounding tissues. Unfortunately, in conventional argon laser photocoagulation visible burns are created, indicating damage to the inner neural retina from the spread of thermal energy beyond the RPE.

Subthreshold diode laser micropulse (SDM) therapy delivers short pulses, which cause less thermal damage. Shorter laser exposure times confine the laser energy to a smaller zone, inflicting less damage on the neural retinal and choriocapillaries. SDM laser has been shown to be as effective as a conventional laser with fewer side effects [28].

7.2.1.2. Steroid injections

Inflammatory factors play an important role in the development of diabetic retinopathy. Upregulation of adhesion molecules in blood vessels leads to leukostasis and the accumulation of macrophages in the retinal vessels. These macrophages release angiogenic growth factors [29] and cytokines which increase vascular permeability. Glucocorticoids block the action of these macrophages and downregulate ICAM-1, which mediates leukocyte adhesion and transmigration [30].

In addition, glucocorticoids alter the composition of endothelial basal membrane by changing the local ratio of two laminin isoforms [31], suppressing basement membrane dissolution, and strengthening tight junctions to limit permeability and leakage that cause macular edema [32]. For this reason, it has long been thought that ocular steroid injections may be beneficial in DME treatment.

Intravitreal triamcinolone acetonide

Triamcinolone acetonide (TA) is a synthetic steroid of the glucocorticoid family with a molecular weight of 434.50. In 2001–2002, the first reports were published of the use of intravitreal injection of triamcinolone acetonide for DME [33,34]. The most common dose used is 4 mg.

Sutter et al. [35] reported in a prospective, double-masked, and randomized trial comparing 4 mg intravitreal TA with sham injection (saline). This study reported that 55% of 33 eyes treated with 4 mg of intravitreal TA improved by 5 or more letters of vision at 3 months compared with 16% of 32 eyes treated with sham injection.

The **DRCR.net** (diabetic retinopathy clinical research network) protocol I [36] studied the use of 4 mg TA combined with macular laser. It found that TA combined with laser significantly improved vision over macular laser alone in patients who had previously undergone cataract surgery. In patients who had not previously undergone cataract surgery TA was much less effective.

Potential side effects of corticosteroid injections include cataract formation and glaucoma. Moreover, as the treatment effect wanes, patients require repeated injections that increase the glaucoma and especially the cataract risk.

Instead of intermittent bolus therapy, it is thought that sustained release of a lower-dose glucocorticoid may lead to greater efficacy with fewer complications. This has led to the development of slow-release steroid implants.

Dexamethasone intravitreal implant

Dexamethasone is a strong synthetic member of the glucocorticoid class of steroid, with an anti-inflammatory and immunosuppressant activity 30 times greater than cortisol and 6 times greater than triamcinolone.

A sustained-release intravitreal dexamethasone (DEX) implant (Ozurdex®, Allergan Inc, Irvine, CA) is biodegradable and is placed in the vitreous cavity using a 22-gauge applicator through a small self-sealing puncture.

Dexmathasone implants have been examined in several large studies; The **PLACID** study [37] compared a DEX implant (0.7 mg) to treatment with focal laser. This 1-year study did not show a statistically significant visual improvement with the DEX implant.

The **MEAD** study [38] combined the results of two multicenter 3-year sham-controlled, masked, randomized clinical studies comparing DEX injection to focal laser treatment. Patients receiving the 0.7 DEX implant required mean of 4.1 injections over 3 years. The average visual improvement with the 0.7 mg DEX implant was +6 letters versus +1 letter with focal laser. Rates of cataract-related adverse events in phakic eyes were 67.9% and 20.4% in the DEX implant 0.7 mg, and sham groups, respectively. Two patients (0.6%) in the DEX implant 0.7 mg group required trabeculectomy for severe glaucoma. Based on the MEAD study, the Food and Drug Administration (FDA) approved DEX implants for use in DME.

Fluocinolone acetonide

Fluocinolone acetonide is a corticosteroid with average mass of 452 Da. ILUVIEN is a non-bioerodable intravitreal implant in a drug delivery system containing fluocinolone acetonide. The fluocinolone acetonide (FA) intravitreal implant [39] is administered in the clinic using a 25-gauge inserter designed to release the drug slowly over 36 months. Unlike the DEX implant, it is not bioerodable.

The FAME studies [40] were two phase 3 clinical trials examining the effect of long-acting fluocinolone acetonide inserts in patients with DME. Patients were randomized in a 2:2:1 ratio to the 0.2 µg per day FA implant, the 0.5 µg per day FA implant, or sham injection (saline). The mean improvement in BCVA letter score between baseline and month 24 was 4.4 and 5.4

in the low- and high-dose groups, respectively, compared with 1.7 in the sham group. Cataract extraction was performed 74.9% of all phakic subjects at baseline in the low-dose insert group and 84.5% in the high-dose insert group compared with 23.1% in the sham group.

Severely elevated intraocular pressure requiring glaucoma surgery occurred in 8.1% of patients in the high dose group, 5.8% of patients in the low dose group, compared only 0.5% in the sham treatment group [40].

This FA implant was approved in Europe (Austria, France, Germany, and Portugal) for the treatment of DME unresponsive to all other therapies. However, it was recently denied approval for this use by the US FDA, due to concerns centering on the high risk of severe glaucoma.

7.2.1.3. Anti-vascular endothelial growth hormone compounds

Vascular Endothelial Growth Hormone (VEGF) is a subfamily of growth factors produced by hypoxic cells that act as signal proteins to stimulate angiogenesis and vascular permeability. One of the main drivers of diabetic eye disease is damage to retinal blood vessels leading to tissue ischemia [41]. Hypoxic cells are then stimulated to release VEGF. Unsurprisingly, elevated levels of VEGF have been demonstrated in the eyes of patients with diabetic retinopathy [42,43]. Elevated VEGF stimulates both retinal vessel proliferation and increased vascular permeability producing the macular edema seen in diabetic eye disease [44].

The injection of anti-VEGF agents to the vitreous is both effective and safe. Adverse ocular effects with an incidence rate of less than 1% and include: cataract formation, retinal detachment, vitreous hemorrhage, and infection. Potential systemic adverse effects include: hypertension, stroke, and myocardial infarction but these are very uncommon [45]. Although there is a theoretical risk for arterial thromboembolic events in patients receiving VEGF-inhibitors by intravitreal injection, the observed incidence rate has been low in all studies and similar to that seen in patients randomized to placebo [1,46].

Over the past 10 years, anti-VEGF agents have become the first line of therapy in treating DME. There are three commercially available anti-VEGF agents: (i) Ranibizumab, (ii) Bevacizumab, and (iii) Aflibercept.

Ranibizumab

Ranibizumab (Lucentis®; Genentech, South San Francisco, California) is a humanized monoclonal antibody fragment directed at all isoforms of VEGF-A. Ranibizumab contains only the Fab fragment of the parental anti-VEGF antibody with weight of 48 kDa. Several large clinical trials have investigated the role of Ranibizumab in the treatment of diabetic macular edema.

READ-2 [47] was a 6-month multicenter trial where patients were randomized in a 1:1:1 fashion to macular laser; monthly Ranibizumab; or a combination of laser and monthly Ranibizumab. At 6 months, the combination therapy and Ranibizumab-only groups gained 3.80 and 7.2 letters at month 6, respectively, compared with no change in the laser only group.

RESTORE [48] was a similar 12-month phase 3 clinical trial which compared Ranibizumab to both laser alone and to laser combined with Ranibizumab. All patients receiving Ranibizumab received three initial consecutive monthly injections followed by pro re nata (PRN, as needed) injections as determined at the monthly examination. At month 12, both the Ranibizumab alone and Ranibizumab with laser groups improved by 6 letters, while the laser alone group remained nearly unchanged. Patients required a mean of seven Ranibizumab injections and the change in vision was statistically significant.

As the data supporting Ranibizumab supplanting laser for primary treatment of center-involving DME grew, many physicians were unsure of the continuing role of focal laser in DME. To answer this among other questions, the **DRCR.net** [49,50] performed a randomized trial which notably compared two methods of combining adjuvant laser with Ranibizumab injections. In one arm of the study (prompt laser), focal laser was given to all the patients at initiation and repeated every 4 months as needed. In the other arm (delayed laser), focal laser could only be added if the edema persisted beyond 24 weeks of monthly Ranibizumab treatment. After 3 years of follow-up, the average gain in the prompt laser group was 7 letters compared with 10 letters in the delayed laser group. Based on these results, it is generally accepted that treatment for center-involving DME should begin with an anti-VEGF agent. Focal laser may be added only if the edema is persistent despite several consecutive anti-VEGF injections. The FDA approved Ranibizumab for treatment of DME in 2012.

Bevacizumab

Bevacizumab (Avastin®; Genentech, South San Francisco, California) is a full-length recombinant humanized monoclonal immunoglobulin G1κ antibody weighing 149 kDa which inactivates all VEGF isoforms. It was FDA-approved in 2004 as a treatment for colon cancer. However, as emerging evidence pointed to VEGF as a central player in DME, ophthalmologists began to use bevacizumab as an "off-label" treatment.

One of the criticisms of Bevacizumab use is that it has not been specifically formulated for ocular use. Bevacizumab is sold in large vials intended for intravenous uses and compounding pharmacies aliquot the medication into prefilled syringes for ocular use. Although there have been case reports of contamination due to this extra step in the preparation process, the safety of Bevacizumab for ocular use has been well established in trials for Age-related Macular Degeneration with a side-effect profile similar to Ranibizumab [51].

Bevacizumab has yet to be approved by the FDA for use in DME. Despite this it is used in many jurisdictions because of its efficacy and its significantly lower cost compared with Ranibizumab. One study [52] estimated the cost of treating DME with Ranibizumab was 20-fold higher than treating with Bevacizumab.

BOLT [53], a 2-year trial comparing bevacizumab monotherapy with focal laser, is the best randomized trial supporting the use of Bevacizumab for center-involving DME. Eighty patients with center-involved DME were randomized to receive either every 6-weekly intravitreal bevacizumab injections (1.25 mg) or focal laser monotherapy.

At 2 years, there was a mean gain of 8.6 letters for Bevacizumab alone compared with a mean loss of 0.5 letters in the laser group.

Aflibercept

Aflibercept (EYLEA®-Regeneron Pharmaceuticals, Tarrytown, New York, NY, and Bayer Healthcare Pharmaceuticals, Berlin, Germany) is a 115-kDa anti-VEGF agent. This protein was developed by combining the extracellular binding domains of VEGF receptors1 and 2 to the Fc segment of human immunoglobulin-G1.Similar to Ranibizumab and Bevacizumab, Aflibercept binds to all isomers of the VEGF-A family.

The phase II **DA VINCI** [54] trial compared two doses of Aflibercept, 0.5 mg and 2.0 mg, to laser treatment. The average improvement in visual acuity at 52 weeks was +11 letters for monthly 0.5 mg, +13 letters for monthly 2.0 mg and −1 letters for laser alone.

A separate arm of this trial received 3 monthly 2 mg doses followed by a scheduled dose every 8 weeks. Patients in this arm received an average of 7.2 injections per year, as compared with over 12 for monthly dosing. The average visual change was +10 letters. Ocular adverse events were consistent with those seen in other trials with anti-VEGF drugs.

The recently completed phase III **VIVID** [55] and **VISTA** [56] trials were similarly designed. Both supported the finding that a schedule of 5 monthly doses of Aflibercept followed by regular bimonthly dosing was of similar efficacy to continuous monthly injections.

In 2014, FDA approved EYLEA for the treatment of diabetic macular edema. The recommended dosage is 2 mg every 2 months, after five initial monthly injections.

Method of administration

The injection procedure should be carried out under aseptic conditions, which includes the use of surgical hand disinfection, sterile gloves, a sterile drape, and a sterile eyelid speculum (or equivalent). Adequate anaesthesia and a broad-spectrum topical microbicide to disinfect the periocular skin, eyelid and ocular surface should be administered prior to the injection, in accordance with local practice.

The injection needle should be inserted 3.5-4.0 mm posterior to the limbus into the vitreous cavity, avoiding the horizontal meridian and aiming toward the center of the globe. The injection volume of 0.05 ml is then delivered.

The use of pre- or postinjection topical antibiotics is not recommended as they have not been shown to alter the infection risk [57].

7.2.2. Nonproliferative diabetic retinopathy treatment

Visual acuity is not usually affected in nonproliferative diabetic retinopathy unless there is damage to the macula in the form of macular edema or ischemia. Ocular treatment at this stage is definitively indicated only if there is evidence of macular disease.

7.2.3. Proliferative diabetic retinopathy treatment

The goal of treatment in proliferative diabetic retinopathy (PDR) is to prevent complications and lower the risk of severe vision loss. The mainstay of treatment for PDR is laser ablation of the peripheral retina where laser burns are placed over the entire retina, sparing the central macula. This treatment is called panretinal photocoagulation (PRP). PRP promotes the regression and arrest of progression of retinal neovascularizations by destroying ischemic retinal tissue and reducing ischemia-driven VEGF production [1,10].

The Diabetic Retinopathy Study (DRS) [25,26] evaluated efficacy of PRP treatment in eyes with advanced NPDR or PDR (DRS Group, 1981). The **DRS** study recommended prompt treatment in eyes with high-risk PDR (defined in section 6.4.3), because these eyes had the highest risk for severe visual loss. PRP treatment in these patients reduced the risk of severe visual loss by 50% over 5 years.

The **ETDRS** study [24,58] found that PRP treatment in eyes with early PDR reduced the risk of progression to high-risk PDR by 50%, and significantly reduced the risk of severe visual loss [24]. Based on these results, PRP treatment should be considered in eyes with any stage PDR especially if there is poor metabolic control, a noncompliant patient, or difficulty in maintaining close follow-up.

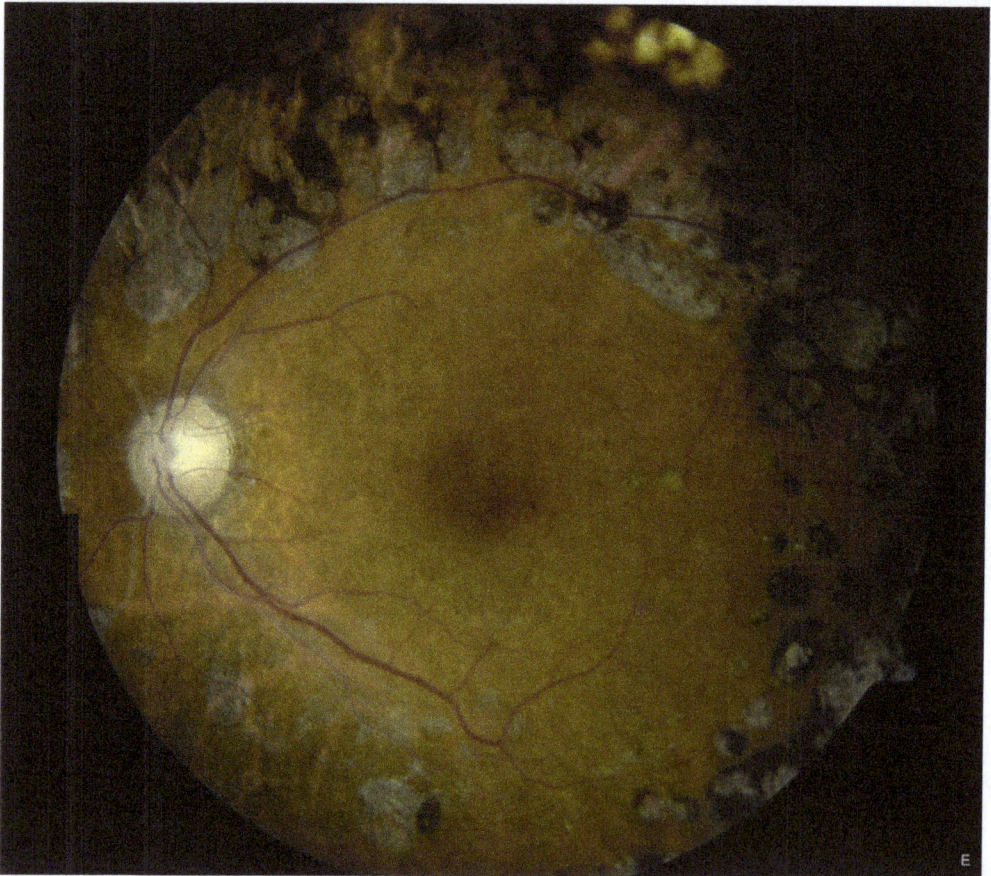

Figure 8. Panretinal photocoagulation: The retinal tissue surrounding the macular region has been ablated using Argon laser. Circular grey-black scars demark areas previously treated with laser burns.

Full PRP treatment as recommended by the **DRS** [25,26] and the **ETDRS** [24,58] includes as many as 5000 laser burns. PRP can be painful and is often performed over several sessions. After the initial treatment course, additional therapy can be applied if there is persistent neovascularization. After treatment, proliferative retinal tissue may regress and contract causing a vitreous hemorrhage or a traction retinal detachment from contracture of fibrovascular tissue. Side effects of PRP treatment also include decreased in night vision, decreased color vision, and loss of peripheral vision [10].

When PDR presents with macular edema, PRP treatment may initially increase the amount of edema [58]. In such case, it is recommended to treat the macular edema with an intravitreal injection before initiating PRP [59,60].

7.2.3.1. Surgery in proliferative diabetic retinopathy

Vitrectomy surgery is most commonly performed in PDR for a dense vitreous hemorrhage causing severe vision loss. If an eye which has not previously undergone PRP develops a significant hemorrhage and vision loss, vitrectomy is recommended when the hemorrhage persists beyond 1–3 months. Patients with vitreous hemorrhage that have preexisting complete PRP may undergo a longer observation period as many patients will have a spontaneous improvement beyond the initial 4 weeks [10,61]. Traction retinal detachment induced by the contraction of neovascular tissue connecting the retinal surface to the vitreous is another serious complication of PDR. If central vision is affected surgery is recommended. However, traction detachments which do not involve the central macula can remain stable for years. Surgery is indicated only when the traction retinal detachment involves or threatens the central macula or if a retinal tear develops [10].

Common complications after vitrectomy include corneal epithelial defects, cataract formation, elevated intraocular pressure, recurrent vitreous hemorrhage, iatrogenic retinal breaks, and rhegmatogenous retinal detachment. The development of these complications can be minimized by meticulous surgical technique and cautious postoperative follow-up.

7.2.3.2. Role of anti-VEGF agents

Several studies have evaluated the efficacy of adjunctive intravitreal anti-VEGF injections in patients with PDR [46]. Adding an anti-VEGF agent to eyes undergoing PRP reduces the risk of a vitreous hemorrhage 12 months after PRP [62]. In eyes with PDR and a dense vitreous hemorrhage, a Bevacizumab injection has been shown to aid significantly in clearing the hemorrhage [63]. This allows PRP to be completed and may reduce the number of patients ending up in surgery.

Bevacizumab has also been shown to enhance retinal surgery in patients with PDR. A single Bevacizumab injection given 1 week before vitrectomy for vitreous hemorrhage, results in decreased bleeding during surgery, decreased operating time, and less postoperative vitreous hemorrhage as compared to vitrectomy [46,64]. As separate study found that a preoperative Bevacizumab injection improved visual acuity 12 months postoperatively compared with vitrectomy alone [62].

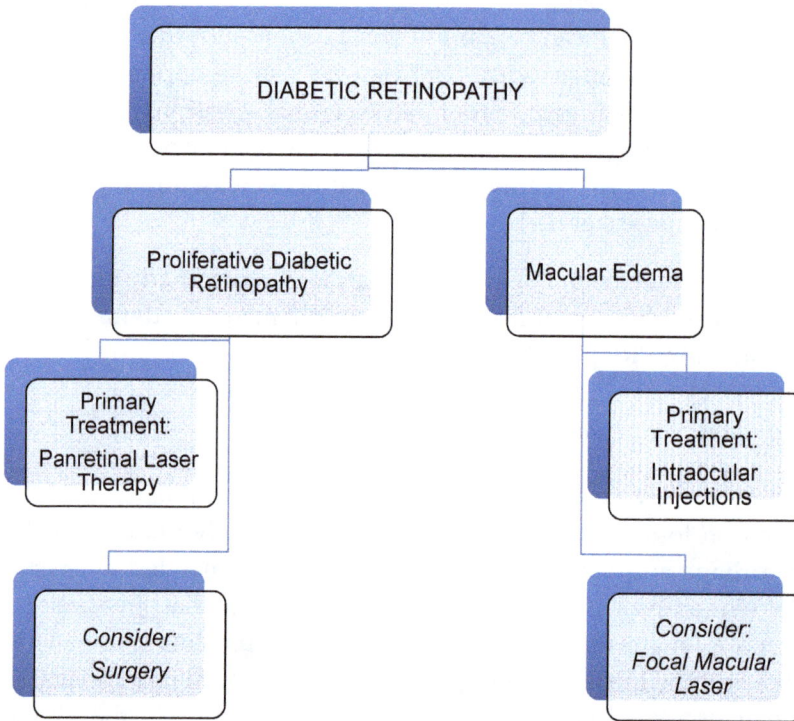

Figure 9. Summary of the two main pathways by which diabetic retinopathy can reduce vision.

7.3. Special considerations

7.3.1. Diabetic retinopathy in pregnancy

In women with preexisting diabetes, pregnancy is considered an independent risk factor for the development and progression of diabetic retinopathy [65]. Most of the progression of diabetic retinopathy in pregnancy occurs by the end of the second trimester. Although regression of retinopathy usually occurs postpartum, there is still an increased risk for progression during the first year postpartum [65]. Risk factors for the development and progression of diabetic retinopathy in pregnancy include longer duration of diabetes before conception, rapid normalization of hemoglobin $A1_C$ at the beginning of pregnancy, poor glycemic control during pregnancy, diabetic nephropathy, high blood pressure, and pree-clampsia [65,66].

Severity of diabetic retinopathy before or at beginning of pregnancy is also a strong predictor of progression of retinopathy during and after pregnancy. The **Diabetes in Early Pregnancy Study** [67] showed that 10.3% of women without diabetic retinopathy and 18.8% with mild NPDR experienced retinopathy progression during pregnancy, and 6.3% of women with mild NPDR progressed to PDR. In women with moderate NPDR, 54.8% suffered retinopathy progression and 29% developed PDR. Overall, progression to sight-threatening diabetic retinopathy, including macular edema and PDR, occurs in 6% of pregnant diabetic women [66].

Progression of retinopathy during pregnancy is probably related to the hypervolemic and hypercoagulable states in pregnancy, as well as elevated pro-inflammatory and angiogenic factor levels. This results in capillary occlusion and leakage-aggravating diabetic retinopathy mechanisms [65,68]. Ideally, good glycemic control and full treatment of preexisting diabetic retinopathy complications should be attained before conception.

All diabetic women who plan pregnancy should be referred by their treating physician to an ophthalmologist. The recommended follow-up of pregnant women with type 1 diabetes includes an ophthalmologic exam at the beginning of pregnancy and during the first trimester. Subsequent follow-up depends on the stage of diabetic retinopathy found on the initial examinations. In women with no retinopathy or very mild NPDR, an ophthalmologic exam is indicated when there are visual complaints. In moderate NPDR, an exam should be done at least once during the second trimester and every 4–6 weeks during the third trimester. In severe NPDR and PDR, close follow-up is needed, and an exam should be done every 4–6 weeks, from the beginning of the second trimester.

Treatment of diabetic retinopathy during pregnancy includes maximal control of both glucose levels and blood pressure [66]. Ocular therapy such as PRP should definitely be performed for PDR and be strongly considered in cases of severe NPDR. Disease progression can be very fast in pregnancy and waiting for PDR to clearly develop may result in severe complications that necessitate invasive surgery. Ocular therapy for PDR and macular edema during pregnancy can include PRP, focal laser, and intravitreal steroid injections. Although there are not much data on the safety of intravitreal injections of anti-VEGF agents during pregnancy, the literature includes some reports on the safe and effective use of Bevacizumab [69].

7.3.2. Cataract surgery in patients with diabetic retinopathy

Cataract development is major factor compromising vision in diabetic patients. Surgery often results in significant vision improvements but these can be mitigated by the progression of diabetic retinopathy and macular edema.

7.3.2.1. Macular edema progression following cataract extraction

Progression of macular edema following cataract extraction can limit the expected improvement in visual acuity from cataract surgery. The reported rates of macular edema following cataract extraction varies from 4% to 70%, depending upon the method used to identify macular edema (angiographic, biomicroscopic, OCT), the cataract extraction technique, and underlying comorbidities [70,71].

The **DRCR.net** [72] conducted a multicenter, prospective, observational study including 293 participants with diabetic retinopathy but without significant macular edema requiring treatment. The authors concluded that in eyes with diabetic retinopathy, the presence of noncentral-involved macular edema immediately prior to cataract surgery, or a history of macular edema treatment may increase the risk of developing central-involving macular edema 16 weeks after cataract extraction.

Topical Nonsteroidal Anti-inflammatory Agents

Controlling postsurgical inflammation is an important factor in preventing macular edema development. Prostaglandin release considerably contributes to fluid leakage from perifoveal capillaries into the extracellular space of the macular region. Multiple studies have reported the benefits of using nonsteroidal anti-inflammatory eye drops pre- and postoperatively to reduce the rate of edema progression [73,74].

Antivascular Endothelial Growth Factor Injections

Recent studies have shown a potential benefit using intravitreal anti-VEGF injections at the end of cataract surgery especially in cases with poorly controlled or refractory macular edema before surgery [46,75,76]. High-risk patients who received intravitreal Bevacizumab or Ranibizumab benefit from better outcomes in terms of visual acuity, macular thickness, and retinopathy progression.

7.3.2.2. Diabetic retinopathy progression following cataract extraction

Controversy exists in the ophthalmic community as to whether cataract surgery potentiates diabetic retinopathy progression. Several studies have reported worsening of diabetic retinopathy and macular edema after surgery [77-80]. Progression was seen during the first year after surgery and was highest in the first 3 months postoperatively. A review of several other studies, especially in the era of cataract surgery using the smaller incision phacoemulsification technique, showed no significant progression of diabetic retinopathy and macular edema after surgery [81,82]. Overall, it is likely that uncomplicated phacoemulsification does not result in a substantially increased risk of the DR progression [83]. The observed rates of progression after uncomplicated, small-incision surgery are similar to the natural course of retinopathy progression over time. The vision improvement and the ability to better visualize the retina to monitor retinopathy progression clearly outweigh the current risks of modern-day cataract extraction and subsequent retinopathy progression over time [83], Overall, diabetics with cataracts benefit from surgery, and improved visual acuity is reported in 92–94% of patients [81]. The combined evidence suggests that in patients with low risk or absent diabetic retinopathy, there is no increased risk of retinopathy progression. However, patients with more advanced retinopathy have an increased risk for retinopathy progression and a worse visual acuity outcome.

7.3.2.3. Summary

A thorough evaluation of patients with diabetes is warranted before cataract surgery. Patients who have severe NPDR or PDR should be considered for PRP treatment prior to cataract removal [84]. Patients with significant macular edema should undergo treatment with a steroid or anti-VEGF agent preoperatively. Ideally, surgery should be delayed until stabilization of retinopathy and macular edema is achieved. In refractory cases, adjunctive therapy with a steroid of anti-VEGF agent at the end of cataract surgery should be considered. Close postoperative follow-up with an ophthalmologist is highly recommended in all patients with preexisting diabetic retinopathy.

8. Schedule for ophthalmologic examinations

Regular ocular examination can detect early ocular disease such as cataracts and glaucoma as well as retinopathy. Diabetic retinopathy in type 1 diabetes is rare during the first 5 years after diagnosis, so the baseline ophthalmologic examination could be extended to 5 years after diagnosis. In children with prepubertal diabetes, the baseline examination should be done at puberty [13].

The timing and frequency of follow-up ocular examinations depends on individual patient's status. In high-risk patients with long-term diabetes and poor systemic risk factor control, annual examinations should be performed even in the absence of retinopathy. In patients with known retinopathy, the examination schedule is based on the degree of retinopathy, and on the patient's compliance and adherence to regular follow-up. In mild NPDR, an examination should be performed every 9–12 months; in moderate NPDR, every 6 months; and in severe NPDR, PDR and CSME follow-up should be even more frequent even in the absence of ongoing treatment [10].

Severity ofRetinopathy	Follow-up Schedule (Months)
None or minimal NPDR	12
Mild NPDR	9-12
Moderate NPDR	6
Severe NPDR	2-4
Non-high-risk PDR	2-4
High-risk PDR	2-4
Diabetic macular edema	1-3

NPDR = non-proliferative diabetic retinopathy; PDR = proliferative diabetic retinopathy

Table 2. Diabetic retinopathy (follow-up recommendations)

9. Conclusion

Diabetes is the leading cause of vision loss in working-age patients, mainly due to diabetic retinopathy. The mainstay in the prevention of disease progression remains optimizing glycemic control and controlling other ancillary risk factors. Laser treatments which prevent vision loss remain an important option for many patients with advanced diabetic retinopathy. Recent advances in medical treatment over the past decade, especially intraocular injections for macular edema, show great promise due to their ability to improve vision. Today, more than ever before, patients with even advanced diabetic eye disease have a good chance of maintaining functional vision for many years provided they undergo proper screening to diagnose complications as they arise. The cost of these new treatments is significant both in financial terms and in terms of patient time investment, as frequent, often monthly, clinic visits are often recommended to optimize results. Additional studies are still needed in order to develop more effective and less costly treatments to further improve the visual prognosis for diabetic patients.

Author details

Efraim Berco[1,2], Daniel Rappoport[1,2], Ayala Pollack[1,2], Guy Kleinmann[1,2] and Yoel Greenwald[1,2*]

*Address all correspondence to: yoel.greenwald@gmail.com

1 Ophthalmology Department, Kaplan Medical Center, Rehovot, Israel

2 Hebrew University and Hadassah Medical School, Jerusalem, Israel

References

[1] Cheung N, Mitchell P,Wong TY. Diabetic Retinopathy. *The Lancet* 2010; 376: 124-36. DOI: 10.1016/S0140-6736(09)62124-3.

[2] Fauci AS, Brownwald E, Kasper DL et al. (Eds.) McGraw-Hill Powers AC. Diabetes Mellitus. *Harrison's Principles of Internal Medicine*. Retrieved from: http://www.access-medicine.com

[3] Thomas D, Graham E. Ocular disorders associated with systemic disease. In: Riordan-Eva P & Whitcher JP (Eds.) *Vaughan & Asbury's General Ophthalmology*, McGraw-Hill,2008. Retrieved from: http://www.accessmedicine.com

[4] Kline LB, Tariq-Bhatti M, Chung SM et al. (Eds.) Section 5: Neuro-ophthalmology. *Basic and Clinical Science Course, -2011,American Academy of Ophthalmology*. American Academy of Ophthalmology.

[5] Leibowitz HM, Krueger DE, Dawber TR et al. The Framingham Eye Study monograph: An ophthalmological and epidemiological study of cataract, glaucoma, diabetic retinopathy, macular degeneration, and visual acuity in a general population of 2631 adults, 1973-1975. *Surv Ophthalmol* 1980; 24:335-610

[6] Obrosova SS, Chung SS, Kador PF. Diabetic cataracts: mechanisms and management. *Diabetes/Metabol Res Rev* 2010:26(3):172-180. DOI:10.1002/dmrr. 1075

[7]   Bobrow JC, Blecher MH, Glasser D et al. (Eds.). Section 11: Lens and cataract. *Basic and Clinical Science Course, 2010-2011, American Academy of Ophthalmology.* Americam Academy of Ophthalmology.

[8]   Purdy EP, Bolling JP, Di-Lorenzo AL et al. (Eds.) Endocrine disorders. In: Section 1: Update on general medicine. *Basic and Clinical Science Course 2010-2011, American Academy of Ophthalmology. 2010;* 189-205, American Academy of Ophthalmology.

[9]   Reidy JJ, Bouchard CS, Florakis GJ et al. (Eds.) Metabolic disorders with corneal changes. In: Section 8: External disease and cornea. *Basic and Clinical Science Course 2010-2011, American Academy of Ophthalmology. 2010;* 307-308. American Academy of Ophthalmology.

[10] Regillo C, Holekamp N, Johnson MW et al. (Eds.) Retinal vascular disease: Diabetic retinopathy. Section 12, Retina and vitreous. *Basic and Clinical Science Course, 2010-2011, American Academy of Ophthalmology.* 2010;109-132. American Academy of Ophthalmology.

[11] Klein R, Knudtson MD, Lee KF et al. The Wisconsin Epidemiologic Study of Diabetic Retinopathy: XXII the twenty-five-year progression of retinopathy in persons with type 1 diabetes. *Ophthalmology* 2008;115(11):1859-1868. doi: 10.1016/j.ophtha. 2008.08.023.

[12] Varma R. From a population to patients: The Wisconsin Epidemiologic Study of Diabetic Retinopathy. *Ophthalmology* 2008; 115(11):1857-1858. DOI: 10.1016/j. ophtha. 2008.09.023.

[13] Raab EL, Aaby AA, Bloom JN et al. (Eds.) Vitreous and retinal diseases and disorders. In: Section 6: Pediatric ophthalmology and strabismus. *Basic and Clinical Science Course 2010-2011, American Academy of Ophthalmology. 2010;* 296-297/ American Academy of Ophthalmology.

[14] DCCT 1995: Progression of retinopathy with intensive versus conventional treatment in the Diabetes Control and Complications Trial. Diabetes Control and Complications Trial Research Group. *Ophthalmology* 1995;102(4): 647-661.

[15] Scanlon PH, Aldington SJ, Stratton IM. Epidemiological issues in diabetic retinopathy. *Middle East Afr J Ophthalmol* 2014;20:293-300. DOI: 10.4103/0974-9233.120007

[16] Price SA, Gorelik A, Wentworth JM et al. Obesity is associated with retinopathy and macrovascular disease in type 1 diabetes. *Obes Res Clin Pract* 2014;8:178-182. DOI: 10.1016/j.orcp.2013.03.007.

[17] Karamanos B, Porta M, Fuller JH et al. Different risk factors of microangionpathy in patients with type 1 diabetes mellitus of short versus long duration. The EURODIAB IDDM complications study. *Diabetologia.* 2000;43:348-355.

[18] DCCT 1997: Clustering of long term complications in families with diabetes in the diabetes control and complications trial. The Diabetes Control and Complications Trial Research Group. *Diabetes* 1997;46(11):1829-1839.

[19] Han L, Zhang L, Zhao J et al. The associations between VEGF gene polymorphisms and diabetic retinopathy susceptibility: a meta-analysis of 11 case-control studies. *J Diabetes Res* 2014;2014 DOI:10.1155/2014/805801.

[20] Gallego PH, Craig ME, Donaghue KC et al. Role of blood pressure in development of early retinopathy in adolescents with type 1 diabetes: Prospective cohort study. *BMJ* 2008;337: 918. DOI: 10.1136/bmj.a918.

[21] Harjutsalo V, Maric C, Groop PH, Finn Diane Study Group. Sex-related differences in the long-term risk of microvascular complications by age at onset of type 1 diabetes. *Diabetologia* 2011;54:1992-1999. DOI: 10.1007/s00125-011-2144-2

[22] DCCT 2000: Effect of pregnancy on microvascular complications in the diabetes control and complications trial. The Diabetes Control and Complications Trail Research Group. *Diabetes Care* 2000; 23(8):1084-1091.

[23] Stirban A, Rosen P, Tschoepe D. Complications of type 1 diabetes: new molecular findings. *Mount Sinai J Med* 2008; 75(4): 328-351. DOI: 10/1002/msj. 20057.

[24] ETDRS 1995: Focal photocoagulation treatment of diabetic macular edema: relationship of treatment effect to fluorescein angiographic and other retinal characteristics at baseline. ETDRS Report 19. Early Treatment Diabetic Retinopathy Study Research Group. *Arch Ophthalmol* 1995;113(9):1144-1155.

[25] DRS 1979: Four risk factors for severe visual loss in diabetic retinopathy. DRS Report 3. Diabetic Retinopathy Study Research Group. *Arch Ophthalmol* 1979; 97(4): 654-655.

[26] DRS 1981: Photocoagulation treatment of proliferative diabetic retinopathy: clinical application of Diabetic Retinopathy Study (DRS) findings. DRS Report 8. Diabetic Retinopathy Study Research Group. *Ophthalmology* 1981;88(7):583-600.

[27] Chaturvedi N, Fuller JH, Aiello LP, EUCLID study Group. Circulating plasma vascular endothelial growth factor and microvascular complications of type 1 diabetes mellitus: the influence of ACE inhibition. *Diabet Med.* 2001;18:288-294.

[28] Venkatesh P, Ramanjulu R, Garg S et al. Subthreshold micropulse diode laser and double frequency neodymium: YAG laser in treatment of diabetic macular edema: a prospective, randomized study using multifocal electroretinography. *Photomed Laser Surg* 2011;29:727-733. DOI: 10.1089/pho.2010.2830.

[29] Ingber DE, Madri JA, Folkman J. A possible mechanism for inhibition of angiogenesis by angiostatic steroids: induction of capillary basement membrane dissolution. *Endocrinology*1986;119(4):1768-1775.

[30] Stokes CL, Weisz PB, Williams SK et al. Inhibition of microvascular endothelial cell migration by beta-cyclodextrin tetradecasulfate and hydrocortisone. *Microvas Res* 1990;40(2):279-284.

[31] Tokida Y, Aratani Y, Morita A et al. Production of two variant laminin forms by endothelial cells and shift of their relative levels by angiostatic steroids. *J Biol Chem* 1990;265(30):18123-9.

[32] Ciulla TA, Harris A, McIntyre N, Jonescu-Cuypers C. Treatment of diabetic macular edema with sustained-release glucocorticoids: intravitreal triamcinolone acetonide, dexamethasone implant, and fluocinolone acetonide implant. *Rev Expert Opin Pharmacother* 2014;15:953-959. DOI: 10.1517/14656566.2014.896899

[33] Jonas JB, Söfker A. Intraocular injection of crystalline cortisone as adjunctive treatment of diabetic macular edema. *Am J Ophthalmol* 2001;132:425-427.

[34] Martidis A, Duker JS, Baumal C et al. Intravitreal triamcinolone for refractory diabetic macular edema. *Ophthalmology* 2002;109:920-927.

[35] Sutter FK, Simpson JM, Gillies MC et al. Intravitreal triamcinolone for diabetic macular edema that persists after laser treatment: three-month efficacy and safety results of a prospective, randomized, double-masked, placebo-controlled clinical trial. *Ophthalmology* 2004;111:2044-2049.

[36] DRCR network 2010a: The Diabetic Retinopathy Clinical Research Network. Randomized trial evaluating Ranibizumab plus prompt or deferred laser or Triamcinolone plus prompt laser for diabetic macular edema. *Ophthalmology* 2010;117(6): 1067-1077. DOI: 10.1016/j.ophtha.2010.02.031.

[37] Callanan D, Gupta S, Boyer D et al. Dexamethasone intravitreal implant in combination with laser photocoagulation for the treatment of diffuse diabetic macular edema. *Ophthalmology* 2013;120;1843-1851. DOI: 10.1016/j.ophtha.2013.02.018

[38] Sadda S, Boyer D, He Yoon Y et al. Safety and efficacy of dexamethasone intravitreal implant in patient with diabetic macular edema: phase III, 3 year, randomized, sham-controlled study [MEAD]. 2014;10:1904-1914. DOI: 10.1016/j.ophtha.2014.04.024

[39] Campochiaro PA, Hafiz G, Shah SM et al. Famous Study Group. Sustained ocular delivery of fluocinolone acetonide by an intravitreal insert. *Ophthalmology* 2010;117(7): 1393-1399. DOI: 10.1016/j.ophtha.2009.11.024

[40] Campochiaro PA, Brown DM, Pearson A et al. Sustained delivery fluocinolone acetonide vitreous inserts provide benefit for at least 3 years in patients with diabetic macular edema. *Ophthalmology* 2012;119(10):2125-2132. DOI: 10.1016/j.ophtha.2012.04.030

[41] Semenza GL. Vascular responses to hypoxia and ischemia. *Arterioscler Thromb Vasc Biol* 2010; 30: 648-652. DOI: 10.1161/ATVBAHA.108.181644

[42] Funatsu H, Yamashita H, Hori S. et al. Angiotensin II and vascular endothelial growth factor in the vitreous fluid of patients with diabetic macular edema and other retinal disorders. *Am J Ophthalmol* 2002;133:537-543.

[43] Aiello LP, Avery RL, Park JE. et al. Vascular endothelial growth factor in ocular fluid of patients with diabetic retinopathy and other retinal disorders. *N Engl J Med* 1994; 331:1480-1487.

[44] Miller JW, Le Couter J, Strauss EC, Ferrara N. Vascular endothelial growth factor a in intraocular vascular disease. *Ophthalmology* 2013; 120: 106-114 DOI: 10.1016/j.ophtha. 2012.07.038

[45] Van der Reis MI, La Heij EC, Schouten JS et al. A systematic review of the adverse events of intravitreal anti-vascular endothelial growth factor injections. *Retina* 2011 Sep;31:1449-1469. DOI: 10.1097/IAE.0b013e3182278ab4.

[46] Nicholson BP, Schachat AP. A review of clinical trials of anti-VEGF agents for diabetic retinopathy. *Graefe's Arch Clin Exper Ophthalmol* 2010; 248(7): 915-930. DOI: 10.1007/ s00417-010-1315-z.

[47] Nguyen QD, Shah SM, Khwaja AA et al. Two-year outcomes of the ranibizumab for edema of the macula in diabetes (READ-2) study. *Ophthalmology* 2010; 117: 2146-2151. DOI: 10.1016/j.ophtha.2010.08.016

[48] Schmidt Erfurth U, Lang GE, Holz FG et al. Three year outcomes of individualized ranibizumab treatment in patients with diabetic macular edema. The RESTORE extension study. Ahead of print. *Ophthalmology* 2014;121:1045-1053. DOI: 10.1016/ j.ophtha.2013.11.041

[49] Elman MJ, Aiello LP, Beck RW et al. Randomized trial evaluating ranibizumab plus prompt or deferred laser or triamcinolone plus prompt laser for diabetic macular edema. *Ophthalmology* 2010;117:1064-1077.e35. DOI: 10.1016/j.ophtha.2014.08.047

[50] Elman MJ, Qin H, Aiello LP et al. Intravitreal ranibizumab for diabetic macular edema with prompt versus deferred laser treatment: three-year randomized trial results. *Ophthalmology* 2012; 119: 2312-2318. DOI: 10.1016/j.ophtha.2012.08.022

[51] Comparison of Age-related Macular Degeneration Treatments Trials (CATT) Research Group, Martin DF,Ferris FL et al. Ranibizumab and bevacizumab for treatment of neovascular age-related macular degeneration: two-year results. *Ophthalmology* 2012;119:1388-1398. DOI: 10.1016/j.ophtha.2012.03.053.

[52] Stefanini FR1, Arevalo JF, Maia M. Bevacizumab for the management of diabetic macular edema. *World J Diabetes* 2013;4:19-26. DOI:10.4239/wjd.v4.i2.19.

[53] Rajendram R, Fraser-Bell S, Kaines A, et al. A 2-year prospective randomized controlled trial of intravitreal bevacizumab or laser therapy (BOLT) in the management of diabetic macular edema: 24-month data: Report 3. *Arch Ophthalmol* 2012;130(8):972–979.

[54] DA VINCI Study Group. One-year outcomes of the DA VINCI study of VEGF trap-eye in eyes with diabetic macular edema. *Ophthalmology* 2012;119(8):1658–1665. DOI: 10.1016/j.ophtha.2012.02.010

[55] Heier J. Intravitreal aflibercept for diabetic macular edema: 12 month efficacy and safety results of phase 3, randomized, controlled VISTA-DME and VIVID-DME studies. 2014.

[56] Diana D. Visual and anatomic outcomes from the VISTA-DME and VIVID-DME studies of intravitreal aflibercept injection in diabetic macular edema patients with and without prior treatment for DME. 2014.

[57] Storey P, Dollin M, Garg SJ et al. Post-Injection Endophthalmitis Study Team. The role of topical antibiotic prophylaxis to prevent endophthalmitis after intravitreal injection. *Ophthalmology* 2014 Jan;121:283-289. DOI: 10.1016/j.ophtha.2013.08.037.

[58] ETDRS 1991: Early photocoagulation for diabetic retinopathy. ETDRS Report 9. Early Treatment Diabetic Retinopathy Study Research Group. *Ophthalmology* 1991;98(5): 766-785.

[59] Silva PS, Sun JK, Aiello LP et al. Role of steroids in the management of diabetic macular edema and proliferative diabetic retinopathy. *Sem Ophthalmol* 2009;24(2):93-99. DOI: 10.1080/08820530902800355.

[60] Mirshahi A, Roohipoor R, Lashay A et al. Bevacizumab-augmented retinal laser photocoagulation in proliferative diabetic retinopathy: a randomized double- masked clinical trial. *Eur J Ophthalmol* 2008;18(2):263-269.

[61] El Annan J, Carvounis PE. Current management of vitreous hemorrhage due to proliferative diabetic retinopathy. *Int Ophthalmol Clin* 2014;54:141-153. DOI: 10.1097/IIO. 0000000000000027.

[62] Martinez-Zapata MJ, Marti-Crvajal AJ, Evans JR et al. Anti-vascular endothelial growth factor for proliferative diabetic retinopathy. 2014;11. DOI: 10.1002/14651858.CD008721.pub2.

[63] Moradian S, Ahmadieh H, Malihi M. et al. Intravitreal Bevacizumab in active progressive proliferative diabetic retinopathy. *Graefe's Arch Clin Exper Ophthalmol.* 2008;246(12):1699-1705. DOI: 10.1007/s00417-008-0914-4.

[64] Ahmadieh H, Shoeibi N, Entezari M, Monshizadeh R. Intravitreal Bevacizumab for prevention of early postvitrectomy hemorrhage in diabetic patients: a randomized clinical trial. *Ophthalmology* 2010; 116:1943-1948. DOI: 10.1016/j.ophtha. 2009.07.001

[65] Shultz KL, Birnbaum AD, Goldsteir DA. Ocular disease in pregnancy. *Curr Opin Ophthalmol* 2005;16(5):308-314.

[66] Vestgaard M, Ringholm L, Laugesen CS et al. Pregnancy-induced sight- threatening diabetic retinopathy in women with type 1 diabetes. *Diabet Med* 2010; 27(4):431-435. DOI: 10.1111/j.1464-5491.2010.02958.x.

[67] Chew EY, Mills JL, Metzger BE et al. Metabolic control and progression of retinopathy. The Diabetic in Early Pregnancy Study. National Institute of Child Health and Human Development. Diabetes in Early Pregnancy Study. *Diabetes Care*1995;18(5): 631-637.

[68] Kastelan S, Tomic M, Pavan J,Oreskovic S. Maternal immune system adaptation to pregnancy – a potential influence on the course of diabetic retinopathy. *Reproduct Biol Endocrinol* 2010;8:124-128. DOI: 10.1186/1477-7827-8-124.

[69] Tarantola RM, Folk JC, Culver Boldt H, Mahajan VB. Intravitreal Bevacizumab during pregnancy. *Retina*. 2010; 30(9): 1405-1411. DOI: 10.1097/IAE.0b013e3181f57d58.

[70] Kim SJ, Equi R, Bressler NM. Analysis of macular edema after cataract surgery in patients with diabetes using optical coherence tomography. *Ophthalmology* 2007 May; 114:881-889.

[71] Ostri C, Lund-Andersen H, La Cour M et al. Phacoemulsification cataract surgery in a large cohort of diabetes patients: visual acuity outcomes and prognostic factors. *J Cataract Refract Surg* 2011;37:2006-2011. DOI: 10.1016/j.jcrs.2011.05.030.

[72] Diabetic Retinopathy Clinical Research Network Authors/Writing Committee, Baker CW, Almukhtar T, Stockdale C et al. Macular edema after cataract surgery in eyes without preoperative central-involved diabetic macular edema. *JAMA Ophthalmol* 2013;131:870-879. DOI: 10.1001/jamaophthalmol.2013.2313.

[73] O'Brien TP. Emerging guidelines for use of NSAID therapy to optimize cataract surgery patient care. *Curr Med Res Opin* 2005 Jul;21:1131-1137.

[74] Singh R, Alpern L, Sager D et al. Evaluation of nepafenac in prevention of macular edema followingcataract surgery in patients with diabetic retinopathy. *Clin Ophthalmol* 2012;6:1259-1269. DOI: 10.2147/OPTH.S31902.

[75] Cheema RA, Al- Mubarak MM, Amin YM et al. Role of combined cataract surgery and intravitreal Bevacizumab injection in preventing progression of diabetic retinopathy; prospective randomized study. *J Cataract Refract Surg* 2009;35:18-25. DOI: 10.1016/j.jcrs.2008.09.019

[76] Chen CH, Liu YC, Wu PC. The combination of intravitreal Bevacizumab and phacoemulsification surgery in patients with cataract and coexisting diabetic macular edema. *J Ocular Pharmacol Therapeut* 2009; 25,83-89. DOI: 10.1089/jop.2008.0068.

[77] Pollack A, Dotan S, Oliver M. Course of diabetic retinopathy following cataract surgery. *Brit J Ophthalmol* 1991;75(1):2-8.

[78] Hauser D, Katz H, Pokroy R. et al. Occurrence and progression of diabetic retinopathy after phacoemulsification cataract surgery. *J Cataract Refract Surg* 2004; 30(2): 428-432.

[79] Jaffe GJ, Burton TC, Kuhn E. et al. Progression of nonproliferative diabetic retinopathy and visual outcome after extracapsular cataract extraction and intraocular lens implantation. *Am J Ophthalmol* 1992; 114(4):448-456.

[80] Hayashi K, Igrarashi C, Hirata A et al. Changes in diabetic macular edema after phacoemulsification surgery. *Eye (London)*. 2009; 23(2): 386-389.

[81] Rashid S, Young LH. Progression of diabetic retinopathy and maculopathy afterphacoemulsification surgery. *Int Ophthalmol Clin/* 2010; 50(1): 155-166. *doi: 10.1097/IIO.0b013e3181c555cf.*

[82] Shah AS, Chen SH. Cataract surgery and diabetes. *Curr Opin Ophthalmol*. 2010:21(1): 4-9. doi: 10.1097/ICU.0b013e328333e9c1.

[83] Haddad NM, Sun JK, Silva PS et al. Cataract surgery and its complications in diabetic patients. *Rev Semin Ophthalmol* 2014;29:329-337. DOI: 10.3109/08820538.2014.959197.

[84] Chew EY, Benson WE, Remaley NA et al. Results after lens extraction in patients with diabetic retinopathy; early treatment diabetic retinopathy study report number 25. Arch Ophthalmol 1999:117(12):1600-1606.

2

Statins in Type 2 Diabetes

Kazuko Masuo

1. Introduction

Cardiovascular disease (CVD) is one of the foremost causes of mortality and is a major contributor to morbidity for individuals with diabetes. Lipids abnormalities play an important role in raising the cardiovascular risk in diabetic and obese individuals. The main components of dyslipidemia in diabetes and metabolic syndrome is documented as small, dense low-density lipoprotein (LDL-cholesterol), the elevation in remnant triglyceride-rich lipoprotein particles, and the low high-density lipoprotein (HDL-cholesterol), which have very powerful atherogenic components.

Diabetes and chronic diseases such as chronic kidney diseases (CKD) were assessed as high-risk for cardiovascular risks by JNC-7, JSH-2009, the Adult Treatment Program III (ATP III)., therefore those conditions require more aggressive control of hypertension and dyslipidemia. [1, 2, 3, 4]. The American Heart Association (AHA) and the American College of Cardiology (ACC) recommended the following four groups of patients should be treated by statins; (1) patients with cardiovascular disease including angina, a previous heart attack or stroke, or other related condition; (2) patients with an LDL cholesterol ≥190 mg/dL; (3) patients with type 2 diabetes aged between 40 and 75 years. They reported that (4) patients with an estimated 10-year risk of cardiovascular diseases including a heart attack or stroke or developing other form of cardiovascular disease of ≥7.5% aged between 40 and 75 years. In addition, both Adult Treatment Program (ATP III) [3] and the American Diabetes Association (ADA) [4] guidelines have identified low-density lipoprotein cholesterol and the first priority of lipid lowering. There is strong evidence from landmark secondary prevention studies, that LDL cholesterol lowering in patients with diabetes leads to significant clinical benefits. Therefore, the benefit of statins on type 2 diabetes has been confirmed. [5]

Assellberg *et al.* [6] found 4 polymorphisms for HDL-cholesterol, 6 polymorphisms of LDL-cholesterol, 10 for total cholesterol, and 4 polymorphisms for triglycerides might be responsible for these lipids' parameters phenotypes in the investigation using 2,000 genes.Genome-wide association studies (GWASs) have shown strong relationships between genetric polymorphisms and lipids levels. Dyslipidemia may have, at least partly, determined genetic backgrounds, and understanding the heritability of dyslipidemia may help to control dyslipidemia.

Dyslipidemia is known as one of the important causes for the atherogenic changes in cardiovascular system, and results in very severe cardiovascular risk. Therefore, diabetes patients with dyslipidemia have much higher prevalence of mortality and morbidity of cardiovascular risks compared to diabetes patients without dyslipidemia. However, there have been a lot of discussions, especially required statins on type 2 diabetes, because statins increase the risk of new-onset type 2 diabetes mellitus [7-9]. Very recent genetic meta-analysis suggested that the increased risk of type 2 diabetes noted with statins is at least partially explained by 3-hydroxy-3-methyl-glutaryl-CoA reductase (HMG-CoA reductase or HMGCR) inhibition [10].

The statins work in the liver to prevent the formation of cholesterol. This class of drugs are most effective at lowering the LDL- cholesterol, but also have modest effects on lowering triglycerides and raising HDL- cholesterol. There are several large cohort studies investigating the effects of statins on cardiovascular risks such as the Scandinavian Simvastatin Survival Study (4S) [11] and the Cholesterol and Recurrent Events (CARE) [12, 13] trial, however, the results are discordant. Some studies showed the drugs to reduce a patient's risk of cardiac events and stroke, outside of their ability to lower cholesterol levels. On the other hand, the statins are known as their side effects including elevation in glucose levels, which is well documented as one of the risk factors for ischemic heart diseases. A number of investigations have shown that people on a high-dose regimen of the cholesterol drug atorvastatin and other cholesterol-lowering drugs may have a slightly increased risk of developing type 2 diabetes, particularly if they have several of the classic diabetes risk factors. Therefore, the American Heart Association (AHA) /The American College of Cardiology (ACC) stated separately the guideline on dyslipidemia in 2013 [14].

This chapter will review *i)* at first, dyslipidemia as a risk factor for cardiovascular diseases, and then *ii)* the benefits and demerits for dyslipidemia treatments in type 2 diabetes using statins based on the data in several large cohort studies. *iii)* Furthermore, the discrepancy, statins can improve dyslipidemia but cannot prevent the new onset of type 2 diabetes, will be discussed.

2. Statins in type 2 diabetes—Friends or Foe?

2.1. Dyslipidemia is one of the criteria of metabolic syndrome, pre-stage of type 2 diabetes

Prevalence of metabolic syndrome has been increasing with prevalence of obesity. The pathophysiology of metabolic syndrome is very complicated, but has been partially understood. It has been well documented metabolic syndrome is an important risk factor for cardiovascular diseases, especially heart diseases including heart failure and ischemic heart disease. Some studies have shown the prevalence of metabolic syndrome in the USA to be an estimated 34% of the adult population [15], and the prevalence increases with age. In addition, weight gain is associated with metabolic syndrome. Central obesity is the most important confounder of metabolic syndrome, therefore, waist circumference may represent the existence of metabolic syndrome (Table 1). Another key confounder of metabolic syndrome is insulin resistance [20, 21]. Hypertensive patients, even they are nonobese, show high prevalence of insulin resistance, and metabolic syndrome coexists. Usually, people with metabolic syndrome has higher risk of developing cardiac events by twice and diabetes by 5 times compared to individuals who do not have metabolic syndrome. Therefore, hypertensive patients, even not obese, with metabolic syndrome have very high risks of cardiac events and diabetes.

	WHO (16)	EGIR (17, 18)	NCEP AT III (Expert Panel on Detection Evaluation and Treatment of High Blood Cholesterol in Adults) (3)	American Heart Association Updated NCEP III (19)
Insulin resistance	Top 25% of population Distribution	Top 25% of population distribution	Not considered	Not considered
Hyperinsulinemia	Not considered	Top 25% of population	Not considered	Not considered
Fasting glucose (mmol/L)	impaired fasting glucose, or impaired glucose tolerance or diabetes	>6.1, but not diabetic	≥6.1	≥5.6 (100 mg/dL) or medications for hyperglycemia
Hypertension (mmHg)	≥160/≥ 90	≥140/≥ 90 or on medications for hypertension	≥130/85	≥130/85 or medications for hypertension
Central obesity	waist/hip ratio >0.9 (men), >0.85 (women) and/or BMI≥30kg/m^2			
Waist circumference (cm)	Not considered	≥94 (men), ≥ 80 (women)	>102 (men), >88 (women)	≥102 (men), ≥88 (women)
HDL-cholesterol (mmol/L)	<1.0 or medications for dyslipidemia	<1.0 or medications for dyslipidemia	<1.07 (40 mg/dL, men), <1.25 (50 mg/dL , women)	<1.07 (40 mg/dL, men) 25 (50 mg/dL, women)
Triglyceride (mmol/L)	<1.0 or medications for Dyslipidemia	>2.0 or medications for dyslipidemia	≥1.695 (150 mg/dL)	≥1.695 (150 mg/dL)
Micro-albuminemia	Present	Not considered	Not considered	Not considered
Criteria	1 of the first two + 2 of other features	2 of other features	3 of above	3 of above

BMI, body mass index; EGIR, European Group of the study of Insulin Resistance; NCEP ATPIII, 3rd Recommendations of the Adult Treatment Panel of the National Cholesterol Education Program; HDL-cholesterol, high-density lipoprotein cholesterol. Values in NECP definition and American Heart Association/Updated NCEP are approximations of values in mg/dL.

Table 1. Criteria for Metabolic Syndrome including Insulin Resistance (11)

In addition, many epidemiological and clinical studies have shown that insulin resistance may lead to dyslipidemia; Dyslipidemia, especially low HDL-cholesterol and high triglycerides are also important criteria with high glucose levels for the metabolic syndrome (Table 1). Carg [22] hypothesized approximately 20 years ago that insulin resistance might cause dyslipidemia in metabolic syndrome. Ruotolo and Howard [23] suggested that hyperinsulinemia as a compensatory mechanisms of insulin resistance leaded to, at first, very low-density of lipoprotein (VLDL) cholesterol overproduction, then the decreased clearance of fasting and postprandial triglyceride rich lipoproteins (TRLs), and the decreased production of HDL particles [23]. In addition, they suggested that increases in TRLs play major role in metabolic syndrome, and elevated VLDL-cholesterol and decreased HDL-cholesterol may be consequence of TRLs elevation. Very recently, the Framingham study [24] supported the close relationship between dyslipidemia and insulin resistance for the onset of coronary heart disease. The incidence of coronary heart disease risk associated with HDL-cholesterol or triglycerides were significantly increased only in the presence of insulin resistance.

2.2. Dyslipidemia is an atherogenic factor

It is well established that elevation of serum LDL is a major cause of atherosclerosis and coronary heart disease (CHD) [25-29]. Many epidemiological studies have shown that elevated LDL cholesterol level is strongly related to future cardiac events [30, 31]. Therefore, LDL-cholesterol can be used as an important predictor for the future cardiac events in cardiac risk assessments (*i.e.* the Framingham Risk Score) [30, 31]. However, it is also known that other serum lipoproteins, such as triglyceride-rich lipoproteins (TRLs), very low-density lipoproteins (VLDL), chylomicrons, and HDL-cholesterol, are involved. In atherogenic dyslipidemia, the pattern of lipoprotein abnormalities or atherogenic lipoprotein phenotype includes elevations of VLDL levels, increased small LDL particles, and low HDL-cholesterol [32, 33]. The abnormalities usually coexist because they have a common metabolic basis. Grundy summarized and figured the relationship insulin resistance, dyslipidemia and coronary heart disease [34]. Besides the multiple mechanisms for atherogenesis accompanying the lipid triad, atherogenic dyslipidemia commonly is associated with several non-lipid risk factors as part of metabolic syndrome (insulin resistance) [35]. In addition, the prothrombotic state may be accompanied by several abnormalities in the coagulation system in metabolic syndrome; most notable are elevations in fibrinogen and plasminogen activator inhibitor-1 (PAI-1). These phenomena might be related to the onset and development of atherogenic damage in vessels

2.3. Statins can improve dyslipidemia in type 2 diabetes, and result in the prevention for coronary heart diseases or other cardiovascular events.

A number of large cohort clinical studies on the efficacy of statins, especially atorvastatin, have been conducted for the primary and secondary prevention of cardiovascular events in adults with, or at risk of, coronary heart disease (CHD). [36, 37] In primary prevention, CARDS (Collaborative Atorvastatin Diabetes Study) [38] showed that atorvastatin 10 mg/day significantly reduced cardiovascular events compared to placebo (relative risk of the composite primary endpoint; acute CHD events, coronary revascularisation, or stroke) by 37% (p = 0.001).

The decrease of cardiovascular events in CARDS study with atorvastatin was similar to those in the ASCOT-LLA (Anglo-Scandinavian Cardiac Outcomes Trial-Lipid Lowering Arm) with atorvastatin [39, 40] and HPS (Heart Protection Study) with simvastatin [41]. However, lipids lowering effects of atorvastatin was observed to be faster compared to simvastatin, 6 months with atorvastatin observed in CARDS [38] versus 15-18 months in simvastatin observed in HPS [41]. The ASCOT-LLA trial [39] conducted in 2,226 hypertensive diabetic patients without previous cardiovascular disease, showed that atorvastatin could decrease the relative risk on primary coronary heart diseases (CHD) by 36% (p=0.0005), and all cardiovascular diseases (CVD) risk by 25% (p = 0.038) compared to placebo. The IDEAL (Incremental Decrease in End Points Through Aggressive Lipid Lowering) [42, 43] and TNT (Treating to New Targets) trials [44, 45] demonstrate that both low (10 mg/day) and high (80 mg/day) doses of atorvastatin reduced the risk of non-fatal myocardial infarction by 17-22% (p < 0.02). [42-45]

Sub-studies of the GREACE (GREek Atorvastatin and Coronary-heart-disease Evaluation) [45-48], TNT (Treating to New Targets) [43, 49-51] and PROVE-IT (PRavastatin Or atorVastatin Evaluation and Infection Therapy) [52-54] trials showed similar results of atorvastatin reduced cardiac events but not only patients without diabetes but also in those with diabetes. Those studies included 15-25% of patients with diabetes.

In the GREACE sub-study, which compared to physicians' standard care [47], atorvastatin significantly reduced the relative risk of total mortality and cardiac moratility and morbidity (coronary mortality, coronary morbidity, and stroke). Furthermore, atorvastatin improved renal function [47] and liver function [46]. Of interest, patients with non-alcoholic fatty liver disease, statins (atorvastatin 24 mg/day) improved liver function, although liver injury was worsen in others without statin treatment for dyslipidemia. This study demonstrated that statin treatment is safe for mild-to-moderate liver injury caused by non-fatty liver disease, and can improve liver injury and reduce cardiovascular morbidity. In addition, statins treatment has benefits for all age groups including old patients. In the older patients, intensive lipids lowering treatments are more effective to reduce cardiovascular risks compared to younger patients when compared to usual lipids lowering treatment. The GREACE study demonstrated that one should not deprive older patients of CVD prevention treatment and lipid target achievement. [48]

Similarly, TNT (Treating to New Targets) trials [49, 50] demonstrate the preventive efficacy of atorvastatin on the reductions of cardiac events in patients with stable CHD. In the TNT sub-study [51] including a total of 9,251 coronary heart disease patients with low-density lipoprotein cholesterol, higher dose of atorvastatin (80 mg/day) over 4.9 years was more effective on the prevention on major cardiovascular events (n=729) such as coronary death, non-fatal myocardial infarction, cardiac arrest, or stroke regardless of fatal or non-fatal, compared to lower dose (10 mg/day). [52] In sub-analysis of TNT trial conducted in 5,584 CHD patients with metabolic syndrome, higher dose of atorvastatin (80mg/day) reduced the major cardio-vascular and cerevrovascular events by 29%. In addition, this sub-study also demonstrated that CHD patients with metabolic syndrome had a 44% greater level of absolute cardiovascular risk compared to those without metabolic syndrome, indicating the clinical feasibility of administering intensive lipid-lowering therapy to CHD patients with metabolic syndrome

[53]. In addition, the other sub-analysis [43] demonstrated even in treatment resistant hypertensive patients, who were at high risk of cardiac events, intensive lipid lowering with atorvastatin 80 mg is associated with a significant reduction in cardiovascular events.

In the PROVE-IT (PRavastatin Or atorVastatin Evaluation and Infection Therapy) sub-study [54, 55], a significantly lower incidence of acute cardiac events was reported in patients with atorvastatin compared to pravastatin (21.1% vs. 26.6%; p = 0.03). Therefore, an absolute risk reduction of 5.5% was associated with atorvastatin therapy [54-56]. Similarly, the IDEAL trial (the Incremental Decrease in End Points through Aggressive Lipid Lowering trial) [57] compared the effects on cardiovascular risks between atorvastatin 80 mg daily versus simvastatin 20-40 mg daily in post-myocardial infarction patients. The IDEAL trial had smaller statistical power due to the smaller number of patients compared to the PROVE-IT study, but longer follow-up (5 years vs. 2 years). Interestingly, decreases in the relative risk of cardiovascular events at 5 years in group with simvastatin was similar to that in the 2-year follow-up with atorvastatin group, and the decreases in the cardiovascular risk maintained consistently from 2 years to 5 years in atorvastatin group. The 2 treatment regimens (atorvastatin versus simvastatin) were well tolerated. These results indicated that patients with recent myocardial infarction should be on intensive statin therapy with atorvastatin and maintain the high dose of atorvastatin as long as possible, over 2 years.

ASPEN (Atorvastatin Study for Prevention of coronary heart disease Endpoints in Non-insulin-dependent diabetes mellitus) [58] in 2,410 type 2 diabetic patients demonstrated that a 29% lower low-density lipoprotein-cholesterol level was seen with atorvastatin than placebo at endpoint (p < 0.0001) over a 4-year period. In sub-analysis in the 505 subjects with prior myocardial infarction or interventional procedure, atorvastatin did not reduce relative risk of a primary end-point (cardiovascular mortality, non-fatal major cardiovascular event, stroke, and unstable angina pectoris, fatal or non-fatal myocardial infaction). Therefore, ASPEN trial failed to confirm the benefit of atorvastatin on cardiocvascular risk in type 2 diabetes [58].

The ALLIANCE (Aggressive Lipid-Lowering Initiation Abates New Cardiac Events) [59-61] and GREACE (GREek Atorvastatin and Coronary-heart-disease Evaluation) [62, 63] trials demonstrated the benefits of treatment with atorvastatin for dyslipidemia compared to usual care with generic statins as the real practical clinic (i.e. simvastatin) in patients with stable CHD. Atorvastatin reduced the risk of non-fatal myocardial infarction by 47-59% (p < 0.0002) compared to usual dyslipidemia therapy with generic statins as a usual community practice in 2008. The MIRACL (Myocardial Ischemia Reduction with Aggressive Cholesterol Lowering) [64, 65], PROVE-IT [54] and IDEAL-ACS (Acute Coronary Syndromes) [57] studies also recommend the benefits of high-dosage atorvastatin therapy started from early phase after the onset of acute coronary syndrome such as within 24-96 hours observed in the MIRACL trial. When compared to placebo, all statins including pravastatin and simvastatin, atorvastatin are effective to reduce the risk of death or major cardiovascular events by 16-18% (p = 0.048). In patients undergoing revascularization procedures, the AVERT (Atorvastatin VErsus Revascularization Treatment) study [66] revealed that administration of atorvastatin 80 mg/day over 18 months had similar benefits on reducing the ischemic cardiac risk to angioplastity plus usual care in low-risk patients with stable coronary artery disease. Furthermore, Arca [62] reviewed that the ARMYDA (Atorvastatin for Reduction in MYocardial DAmage during angioplasty) and ARMYDA-3 trials showed atorvastatin's benefits on myocardial infaction patients; Atorvastatin 40 mg/day over 7 days before coronary intervention significantly reduced the risks of myocardial ischemic damage (ARMYDA), post-procedural acute myocardial infarction (ARMYDA) and atrial fibrillation (ARMYDA-3) versus placebo. In addition, it has been observed that post-myocardial infactionm patients without atorvastatin have significantly higher C-reactive protein levels and higher prevalence of the combined incidence of cardiovascular events (death, MI and target segment revascularization during the 6-month follow-up). In addition, the ATTEMP study (Assessing The Treatment Effect in Metabolic syndrome without Perceptible diabetes) [67] showed atorvastatin improved renal function and reduced serum uric acid levels in metabolic syndrome without cardiovascular diseases. These changes were more prominent in stage 3 chronic kidney diseases patients and might have contributed to the reduction in cardiovascular risk and clinical events.

Overall, therefore, the marked efficacy of atorvastatin in the primary and secondary prevention of cardiovascular events were provided in many large cohort trials not only in relative healthy individuals, but also in diabetes or post-myocardial infarction patients, and the effects were stronger than usual statins such as simvastatin. Atorvastatin has in general cardiovascular disease management including improving renal function, and liver injury with non-alcoholic fatty liver, suggests even greater potential clinical utility for the drug in some clinical settings. [37, 66] The results from the meta-analysis using 31 randomized studies compared statins and placebo or other statins showed in patients with CVD, (or at risk of CVD), statin reduced relative risk of all cause mortality, cardiovascular mortality, coronary heart disease mortality and fatal myocardial infarction, but did not reduce the risk of fatal stroke. Statin could not reduce relative risk of morbidity of non-fatal stroke, non-fatal myocardial infarction, transient ischemic attack (TIA), unstable angina, and coronary revascularization.

The differentiations on the clinical efficacy between statins; atorvastatin, fluvastatin, pravastatin and simvastatin, are almost impossible from the previous large clinical studies, however, there is some evidence from direct comparisons between statins to suggest that atorvastatin may be more effective than pravastatin in patients with symptomatic coronary heart diseases, although there is limited evidence for the effectiveness of statins in different subgroups [67].

2.4. Statins may improve renal function

The comparisons analysis related to renal function [43] from clinical trials with data from 149,882 patient-years of follow-up failed to show an association between high-potency statins and risk of acute kidney injury with statins (10,345 patients on atorvastation, 10-80 mg/day) compared with controls (placebo, 8,945 patients with placebo). In addition, there were no differences in effects on renal function between high-dose versus low-dose. This comparison was performed in the 24 placebo-controlled trials including IDEAL [57], TNT [47], CARDS [69, 70], ASPEN (The Atorvastatin Study for Prevention of coronary heart disease Endopoints in Non-diabeties mellitus) [58], SPARCL (The Stroke Prevention by Aggressive Reduction in Cholesterol Levels) [43, 71], and other large study using placebo with 10,345 patients with atorvastatin and 8945 patients with placebo. [43]

The TNT trial in 10,001 CHD patients with and without pre-existing chronic kidney diseases demonstrated efficacy of atorvastatin (80 mg/day) on reduction of CHD risk as well as improving renal function in both with and without pre-existing renal injury patients. No difference in the incidence of renal-related serious adverse events were observed at 120 days (0.04% in atorvastatin; 0.10% in placebo, p = 0.162) [50, 51]. Similarly, the use of a high-potency statin regimen did not increase the risk of kidney injury was observed in 2 large randomized trials of statin therapy in patients with acute coronary syndrome; PROVE IT-TIMI 22 [50, 55] (atorvastatin 80 mg/day) including 4,162 patients, and A-to-Z trial (pravastatin 40 mg/day for 1 month + simvastatin 80 mg/day after 1 month) including 4, 497 patients. [72] As mentioned in the previous section, the ATTEMP (Assessing the treatment Effect in Metabolic syndrome without Perceptible diabetes) study [67] showed that multifactorial intervention in patients with metabolic syndrome without established CVD improved renal function and reduced serum uric acid levels. Of importance, these changes were more prominent in stage 3 chronic kidney diseases patients. PROVE-IT-TIMI 22 sub-study [73] used urinary albumin excretion as an index of renal injury, showed no significant change in urinary albumin concentration from enrollment to end of study in either the standard (pravastatin 40 mg/day) or intensive (atorvastatin 80 mg/day) statin therapy groups in an acute coronary syndrome in statin treated patient. [52] Microalbuminuria may reflect traditional cardiovascular risk factor burden and offer little prognostic information independent of those factors. [52]

2.5. Cost-effectiveness

Cost-effectiveness between statins has been compared in several studies such as the Aggressive Lipid-lowering Initiation Abates New Cardiac Events study (ALLIANCE study) [73], and those observations showed the advantage of atorvastatin in high-risk CVD patients [68] and type 2 diabetes patients [74]. Despite the non-adherence levels observed in actual practice, statin treatment is cost-effective for primary prevention in patients newly diagnosed with type 2 diabetes. Because of large differences in cost-effectiveness according to different risk and age groups, the efficiency of the treatment could be increased by targeting patients with relatively higher cardiovascular risk and higher ages [74]. When the efficacy and cost-effectiveness were compared between rosuvastatin, atorvastatin, pravastatin and simvastatin, rosuvastatin therapy in commonly prescribed doses is most effective for improving hypercholesterolemia and most cost effective in diabetic patients with and without metabolic syndrome. [75] The PROVE IT trial [76] demonstrated that atorvastatin 80 mg/day has stronger efficacy on reducing cardiovascular events compared to pravastatin 40 mg/day in patients with acute coronary syndrome. Genetic investigations in PROVE-IT sub-study showed that the preva-lence of event reduction was greater in carriers of the Trp719Arg variant in kinesin family member 6 protein (KIF6) than in non-carriers. Parthan et al. [76] assessed the cost effectiveness of testing for the KIF6 variant followed by targeted statin therapy (KIF6 Testing) versus not testing patients, and they found that cost-effectiveness is sensitive to the price of generic atorvastatin and the effect on adherence of knowing KIF6 carrier status.

2.6. The JUPITER trial and meta-analyses show statins increase the risk of new onset of type 2 diabetes

Statins are known as well-tolerated and very rare adverse events reported. Side effects of statins are very rare but still exist such as elevations of liver enzymes, muscle aches, and very rarely, rhabdomyolysis [76]. If people have adverse events, discontinuation is primary as usual procedure to resolve these adverse events similarly to other any medications.. Recently, debate has focused on the possible negative long-term effects of statin treatment on cognitive decline, and the incidence of cancer [78]. Some investigators have documented that statins affect the risk of developing cancer, when they are taken at low doses for managing hypercholestero-laemia. There is some possibility of an increased cancer risk in elderly patients associated with hydrophilic statin use. On the other hand, some recent studies have shown the benefits of statins in modifying the prognosis of cancer, and the decreases in the risks of certain cancers, such as gastric, oesophageal, liver, colorectal and advanced/aggressive prostate cancer. In addition, Jukema *et al.* [78] reported that there was no increased risk of cognitive decline or cancer with statin use. However, regarding the relations between statins and cancer, results remain controversial. Further investigations will be necessary to clarify.

Since the report of the new onset of diabetes during rosuvastatin treatment, as an unexpected finding in the JUPITER trial [7], safety concerns on abnormal glucose metabolisms related to statins have emerged in 2012. The possible association of diabetes with statin therapy has been discussed over several years, but statins' effects on reducing of cardiovasculoar risk has been overweighted than the new onset of diabetes or glucose metabolism impairement. In addition, guidelines of the American Diabetes Association [3], American Heart Association [1, 14], and American Copllege of Cardiology [14] have shown the same direction of overweighting on dyslipidemia control. In addition, several studies and meta-analysis data have shown that statin use is related to a small increased risk of type 2 diabetes mellitus. The JUPITER (Justifi-cation for the Use of Statins in Prevention: an Intervention Trial Evaluating Rosuvastatin) trial [79-81] demonstrated new onset of diabetes, although rosuvastatin reduces cardiovascular events and all-cause mortality and concomitant evidence of moderate chronic kidney diseases. The JUPITER finding on impairement of glucose metabolisms was the first data showing the strong relationship between statins and the new onset of diabetes. The JUPITER trial [78, 80]was conducted in 17,603 men and women without histories of cardiovascular diseases or diabetes with randomized, double blind design to evaluate the efficacy of rosuvastatin 20 mg/day over 5 years. In this trial, the participants who had diabetes risk factor (n=11,508), showed developing diabetes more frequently than those without a diabetic risk factor (n=6,095). In individuals with diabetic risk factors, rosuvastatin decreased the cardiovascular risks such as the primary endpoint by 39%, venous thrombosis by 36%, and total mortality by 17%, but increased diabetes risk by 28 %. On the other hand, in the participants without diabetic risk factors, all parameters decreased significantly with larger drops compare dto those with diabetic risk factors (primary endpoint by 52%; venous thrombosis by 53%; total mortality by 22 %). And, importantly, no elevations in the new onset of diabetes or impairment of glucose metabolism were observed. These results suggested that statins may have more stronger benefits on reduction of cardiovascular risks and glucose metabolisms in individuals without diabetes compared to those with diabetes. When compared to placebo, the onset of diabetes needed longer duration by 5,4 weeks in rosuvastatin (rosuvastatin, 84.3 weeks vs placebo, 89.7 weeks). The benefits on cardiovascular risk and total mortality in rosuvastatin group were greater than the hazard of the new onset of diabetes [7].

Furthermore, three recent meta-analyses of large-scale placebo-controlled and standard care-controlled trials [82] showed approximately more than 10% increased risk for incident diabetes associated with statin therapy. [83, 84]

On the other, recently the post hoc analysis of ATTEMPT study assesses the incidence of new-onset diabetes over 3.5 years in patients with metabolic syndrome observed no differences in the new onset of diabetes in patients with statins (statins, 0.83 vs. placebo, 1.00/100 patient-years) from the general population [67, 85], and no differences in the new onset of diabetes between individuals with and without diabetic risk factors [84]. New-onset diabetes incidence and CVD events were negligible and not different from what is expected in the general population. [85]

Park *et al.* [9] analysed the linkage of statins and the new-onset diabetes using meta-analysis in published large cohort studies in MEDLINE from 2000 to October 2013 with the following MESH terms and text key words alone or in combination were included: 3-hydroxy-3-methylglutaryl coenzyme A reductase inhibitors, HMG-CoA reductase inhibitors, statins, incident diabetes, new-onset diabetes, insulin resistance, impaired insulin secretion, meta-analysis, cohort study, and observational study written in English. Results of observational studies and meta-analyses show association of incident diabetes with statin use in patients with concomitant risk factors for diabetes. They concluded a possible association between statin use and incident diabetes in patients with underlying diabetes risk factors in available clinical data. Although study data may be insufficient to change the current practice paradigm, clinicians should vigilantly monitor for incident diabetes in patients on statins. Patients with a low risk of CVD and high risk of diabetes should reconsider statin use and focus on lifestyle management. Each statins has different effects on glucose metabolisms, and women and elderly persons are known at higher risk of diabetes. Therefore, various confounders related to adverse events, especially glucose metabolisms, should be considered

Muscoqiuri, *et al.* [86] discussed the effects of statins on insulin sensitivity or insulin secretion, because statins deteriorates glycemic control may accelerate progression to diabetes via molecular mechanisms that impact insulin sensitivity and secretion. The weight of clinical evidence suggests a worsening effect of statins on insulin resistance and secretion, but basic science studies could not find a clear molecular explanation from searches of computerized databases, providing conflicting evidence regarding both the beneficial and the adverse effects of statin therapy on insulin sensitivity.

A number of meta-analyses conducted in recent years have demonstrated that the association is real but causality has not yet been proved [8]. And the underlying mechanisms for this association remain unclear.

In summary, although many clinical studies have demonstrated that statins worsen glucose metabolism or cause the new onset of diabetes, the cardiovascular benefits of statin therapy overweigh the risk of impairment of glucose metabolism. Clinical practice for statin therapy should not be changed on the basis of the most recent Food and Drug Administration informational warnings in 2012. Therefore, the data suggest the need to treat dyslipidemia and to make patients aware of the possible risk of developing type 2 diabetes or, if they already are diabetic, of worsening their metabolic control.

3. Conclusions

In 2014, Simic and Reiner [87] summarized benefits and side effects of stastins as follow; 1) reduction in cardiovascular mortality and morbidity even in patients with very high risk of cardiovascular disease; 2) myopathy and rhabdomyolysis as most important side effects; 3) liver injury as a side effects, which occurs occasionally but is reversible. On the other hand, statins also improve hepatic steatosis and liver injury in fatty liver diseases; 4) similarly, renal injury as a side effect, but also statins showed protective effects on renal injury [69] and majority of data have shown the beneficial effects on renal function [33, 50-53, 67. 72]. 5) statins increase the incidence of type 2 diabetes, especially in individuals with diabetic risk factors [78]. But the cardiovascular benefits of such a treatment by far exceed this risk. Therefore, currently many guidelines for treatments for dyslipidemia, diabetes concluded that the cardiovascular benefits of statins by far outweight non-cardiovascular harms in patients with cardiovascular risk. However, it should be needed to treat dyslipidemia and to make patients aware of the possible risk of developing type 2 diabetes or, if they already are diabetic, of worsening their metabolic control.

Author details

Kazuko Masuo*

Address all correspondence to: kazuko.masuo@bakeridi.edu.au

Baker IDI Heart & Diabetes Institute, Melbourne, Victoria, Australia

The author declares no conflict of interest.

References

[1] US Department of Health and Human Services. National Institutes of Health National Heart, Lung, and Blood Institute. JNC 7 Express. The Seventh Report of Joint National Committee on Prevention, Detection, Evaluation, and Treatment of High Blood Pressure. 2003. http://www.nhlbi.nih.gov/files/docs/guidelines/express.pdf.

[2] Ogihara T, Kikuchi K, Matsuoka H, Fujita T, et al. Japanese Society of Hypertension Committee. The Japanese Society of Hypertension Guidelines for the Management of Hypertension (JSH 2009). Hypertens Res. 2009 Jan;32(1):3-107.

[3] Third report of the National Cholesterol Education Program (NCEP) Expert Panel on Detection, Evaluation, and Treatment of High Blood Cholesterol in Adults (Adult Treatment Panel III) final report. Circulation. 2002; 106: 3143-3121.

[4] American Diabetes Association. Standards of medical care in diabetes—2013. Diabetes Care. 2013 Jan;36 Suppl 1:S11-66. doi: 10.2337/dc13-S011

[5] Carmena R, Betteridge DJ. Statins and diabetes. Semin Vasc Med. 2004; 4: 321-332.

[6] Asselbergs FW, Guo Y, van Iperen EP, Sivapalaratnam S, Tragante V, Lanktree MB, et al. Large-scale gene-centric meta-analysis across 32 studies identifies multiple lipid loci. Am J Hum Genet. 2012; 91: 823-838. doi: 10.1016/j.ajhg.2012.08.032.

[7] Ridker PM, Pradhan A, MacFadyen JG, Libby P, Glynn RJ. Cardiovascular benefits and diabetes risks of statin therapy in primary prevention: an analysis from the JUPITER trial. Lancet. 2012; 380: 565-571. doi: 10.1016/S0140-6736(12)61190-8.

[8] Aiman U, Najmi A, Khan RA. Statin induced diabetes and its clinical implications. J Pharmacol Pharmavother. 2014; 5: 181-184. doi: 10.4103/0976-500X.136097.

[9] Park ZH, Juska A, Dyakov D, Patel RV. Statin-associated incident diabetes: a literature review. Consul Pharm. 2014; 29: 317-334. doi: 10.4140/TCP.n.2014.317.

[10] Swerdlow DI, Preiss D, et al. HMG-coenzyme A reductase inhibition, type 2 diabetes, and bodyweight: evidence from genetic analysis and randomised trials. Lancet. 2014 Sep 24. pii: S0140-6736(14)61183-1. doi: 10.1016/S0140-6736(14)61183-1.

[11] Huskey J, Lindenfeld J, Cook T, Targher G, Kendrick J, Kjekshus J, Pedersen T, Chonchol M. Effect of simvastatin on kidney function loss in patients with coronary heart disease: findings from the Scandinavian Simvastatin Survival Study (4S). Atherosclerosis. 2009; 205: 202-206. doi: 10.1016/j.atherosclerosis.2008.11.010.

[12] Sheng X, Murphy MJ, MacDonald TM, Wei L. The comparative effectiveness of statin therapy in selected chronic diseases compared with the remaining population. BMC Public Health. 2012; 12: 712. doi: 10.1186/1471-2458-12-712.

[13] Miyazaki T, Chiuve S, Sacks FM, Ridker PM, Libby P, Aikawa M. Plasma pentraxin 3 levels do not predict coronary events but reflect metabolic disorders in patients with coronary artery disease in the CARE trial. PLoS One. 2014; 9: e94073. doi: 10.1371/journal.pone.0094073. eCollection 2014.

[14] Stone NJ, Robinson J, et al. Expert panel Members, and ACC/AHA Task Force Members. 2013 ACC/AHA Guideline on the Treatment of Blood Cholesterol to Reduce Atherosclerotic Cardiovascular Risk in Adults. A Report of the American College of Cardiology/American Heart Association Task Force on Practice Guidelines. at VA

MED CTR BOISE on December 24, 2014. http://circ.ahajournals.org/ (Download at VA MED CTR BOISE on December 24 2014).

[15] Ford ES, Giles WH, Dietz WH. Prevalence of metabolic syndrome among US adults: findings from the third National Health and Nutrition Examination Survey. JAMA 2002; 287: 356–359. doi:10.1001/jama.287.3.356. PMID 11790215.

[16] Alberti KG, Zimmet PZ. Definition, diagnosis and classification of diabetes mellitus and its complications. Part 1: diagnosis and classification of diabetes mellitus provisional report of a WHO consultation. Diabet Med. 1998; 15: 539-553.

[17] Balkau B, Charles MA. Comment on the provisional report from the WHO consultation. European Group for the study of Insulin Resistance (EGIR). Diabet Med. 1999; 16: 442-443.

[18] Balkau B, Charles MA, Drivsholm T, et al. European Group for the study of Insulin Resistance (EGIR). Frequency of the WHO metabolic syndrome in European Cohorts, and an alternative definition of an insulin resistance syndrome. Diabetes Metab. 2002; 28: 364-376.

[19] Grundy SM, Brewer HB, Cleeman JI, Smith SC Jr, Lenfant C, The American Heart association, the National Heart, Lung, and Blood Institute : Definition of metabolic syndrome: Report of the National Heart, Lung, and Blood Institute/American Heart association conference on scientific issues related to definition. Circulation. 2004; 109: 433-438.

[20] DeFronzo RA, Ferrannini E. Insulin resistance. A multifaceted syndrome responsible for NIDDM, obesity, hypertension, dyslipidemia, and atherosclerotic cardiovascular disease. Diabetes Care. 1991; 14: 173-194.

[21] Ferrannini E. Definition of intervention points in prediabetes. Lancet Diabetes Endocrinol. 2014; 2: 667-675. doi: 10.1016/S2213-8587(13)70175-X.

[22] Carg A. Insulin resistance in the pathogenesis of dyslipidemia. Diabetes Care. 1996; 19: 387-389.

[23] Robins SJ, Lyass A, Zachariah JP, Massaro JM, Vasan RS. Insulin resistance and the relationship of a dyslipidemia to coronary heart disease: The Framingham Heart Study. Arterioscler Thromb Vasc Biol. 2011; 31: 1208-1214.

[24] Ruotolo G, Howard G. Dyslipidemia in the metabolic syndrome. Curr Cardiolo Rep. 2004; 4: 494-500]

[25] Expert Panel on Detection, Evaluation, and Treatment of High Blood Cholesterol in Adults. National Cholesterol Education Program: second report of the Expert Panel on Detection, Evaluation, and Treatment of high blood cholesterol (Adult Treatment Panel II). Circulation. 1994; 89: 1329-1445.

[26] Stamler J, Wentworth D, Neaton JD. Is the relationship between serum cholesterol and risk of premature death from coronary heart disease continuous and graded?

Findings in 356,222 primary screenees of the Multiple Risk Factor Intervention Trial (MRFIT). JAMA. 1986; 256: 2823-2828.

[27] Scandinavian Simvastatin Survival Study Group. Randomised trial of cholesterol lowering in 4444 patients with coronary heart disease: the Scandinavian Simvastatin Survival Study (4S). Lancet. 1994; 344: 1383-1389.

[28] The Long-Term Intervention with Pravastatin in Ischaemic Disease (LIPID) Study Group. Prevention of cardiovascular events and death with pravastatin in patients with coronary heart disease and a broad range of initial cholesterol levels. N Engl J Med. 1998; 339: 1349-1357.

[29] Shepherd J, Cobbe SM, Ford I, et al, for the West of Scotland Coronary Prevention Study Group. Prevention of coronary heart disease with pravastatin in men with hypercholesterolemia. N Engl J Med. 1995; 333: 1301-1307.

[30] hah RV, Goldfine AB. Statins and risk of new-onset diabetes mellitus. Circulation. 2012; 126: e282-e284. doi: 10.1161/CIRCULATIONAHA.112.122135

[31] Cobain M, Massaro J, Kannel W. General cardiovascular risk profile for use in primary care: the Framingham Heart Study. Circulation. 2008;117:743–753.

[32] Grundy SM. Atherogenic dyslipidemia: lipoprotein abnormalities and implications for therapy. Am J Cardiol. 1995; 75: 45B-52B.

[33] Grundy SM. Small LDL, atherogenic dyslipidemia, and the metabolic syndrome. Circulation. 1997; 95: 1-4.

[34] Grundy SM. MedScape Diabetes & Endocrinology. http://www.medscape.com/view-article/412684_2

[35] Grundy SM. Hypertriglyceridemia, atherogenic dyslipidemia, and the metabolic syndrome. Am J Cardiol. 1998; 81: 18B-25B.

[36] Ward S, Lloyd JM, Pandor A, Holmes M, Ara R, et al. A systemic review and economic evaluation of statins for the prevention of coronary events. Health Technol Assess. 2007; 11: 1-160, iii-iv.

[37] Arca M. Ateovastatin efficacy in the prevention of cardiovascular events in patients with diabetes mellitus and/or metabolic syndrome. Drugs 2007; 67 Suppl 1: 43-54.

[38] Newman CB, Szarek M, Colhiun HM, Betteridge DJ, et al. The safety and tolerability of atorvastatin 10 mg in the Collaborative Atorvastatin Diabetes Study (CASRDS). Diab Vasc Dis Res. 2008; 5: 177-183. doi: 10.3132/dvdr.2008.029.

[39] Sever PS, Chang CL, Gupta AK, Whitehouse A, Poulter NR; ASCOT Investigators. The Anglo-Scandinavian Cardiac Outcomes Trial: 11-year mortality follow-up of the lipid-lowering arm in the U.K. Eur Heart J. 201; 32: 2525-2532. doi: 10.1093/eurheartj/ehr333.

[40] Chapman N, Chang CL, Caulfield M, Dahlöf B, Feder G, Sever PS, Poulter NR. Ethnic variations in lipid-lowering in response to a statin (EVIREST): a substudy of the Anglo-Scandinavian Cardiac Outcomes Trial (ASCOT). Ethn Dis. 2011; 21: 150-157.

[41] Heart Protection Study Collaborative Group, Bulbulia R, Bowman L, Wallendszus K, Parish S, et al. Effects on 11-year mortality and morbidity of lowering LDL cholesterol with simvastatin for about 5 years in 20,536 high-risk individuals: a randomised controlled trial. Lancet. 2011; 378: 2013-2020. doi: 10.1016/S0140-6736(11)61125-2.

[42] Arsenault BJ, Boekholdt SM, Hovingh GK, Hyde CL, et al. TNT and IDEAL Investigators.The 719Arg variant of KIF6 and cardiovascular outcomes in statin-treated, stable coronary patients of the treating to new targets and incremental decrease in end points through aggressive lipid-lowering prospective studies. Circ Cardiovasc Genet. 2012; 5: 51-57. doi: 10.1161/CIRCGENETICS.111.960252.

[43] Bangalore S, Fayyad R, Hovingh GK, Laskey R, et al. Treating to New Targets Steering Committee and Investigators. Statin and the risk of renal-related serious adverse events: Analysis from the IDEAL, TNT, CARDS, ASPEN, SPARCL, and other placebo-controlled trials. Cardiol. 2014; 113: 2018-2020. doi: 10.1016/j.amjcard.2014.03.046.

[44] Arsenault BJ, Boekholdt SM, Mora S, DeMicco DA, et al. Impact of high-dose atorvastatin therapy and clinical risk factors on incident aortic valve stenosis in patients with cardiovascular disease (from TNT, IDEAL, and SPARCL). Am J Cardiol. 2014; 113:1378-1382. doi: 10.1016/j.amjcard.2014.01.414.

[45] Athyros VG, Tziomalos K, Gossios TD, Griva T, et al. GREACE Study Collaborative Group. Safety and efficacy of long-term statin treatment for cardiovascular events in patients with coronary heart disease and abnormal liver tests in the Greek Atorvastatin and Coronary Heart Disease Evaluation (GREACE) Study: a post-hoc analysis. Lancet. 2010; 376: 1916-1922. doi: 10.1016/S0140-6736(10)61272-X.

[46] Athyros VG, Kakafika AI, Papageorgiou AA, Paraskevas KI, et al. Effects of statin treatment in men and women with stable coronary heart disease: a subgroup analysis of the GREACE Study. Curr Med Res Opin. 2008; 24:1593-1599. doi: 10.1185/03007990802069563.

[47] Athyros VG, Kakafika AI, Papageorgiou AA, Pagourelias ED, et al. Statin-Induced Increase in HDL-C and Renal Function in Coronary Heart Disease Patients. Open Cardiovasc Med J. 2007; 1: 8-14. doi: 10.2174/1874192400701010008.

[48] Athyros VG, Katsiki N, Tziomalos K, Gossios TD, et al. GREACE Study Collaborative Group. Statins and cardiovascular outcomes in elderly and younger patients with coronary artery disease: a post hoc analysis of the GREACE study. Arch Med Sci. 2013; 9: 418-426. doi: 10.5114/aoms.2013.35424.

[49] Ong KL, Waters DD, Messig M, DeMicco DA, Rye KA, Barter PJ. Effect of change in body weight on incident diabetes mellitus in patients with stable coronary artery dis-

ease treated with atorvastatin (from the treating to new targets study). Am J Cardiol. 2014; 113: 1593-1598. doi: 10.1016/j.amjcard.2014.02.011.

[50] LaRosa JC, Deedwania PC, Shepherd J, Wenger NK, Greten H, DeMicco DA, Breazna A; TNT Investigators. Comparison of 80 versus 10 mg of atorvastatin on occurrence of cardiovascular events after the first event (from the Treating to New Targets [TNT] trial). Am J Cardiol. 2010; 105: 283-287. doi: 10.1016/j.amjcard.2009.09.025.

[51] Ho JE, Waters DD, Kean A, Wilson DJ, Demicco DA, Breazna A, Wun CC, Deedwania PC, Khush KK. TNT Investigators. Relation of improvement in estimated glomerular filtration rate with atorvastatin to reductions in hospitalizations for heart failure (from the Treating to New Targets [TNT] study). Am J Cardiol. 2012; 109:1761-1766. doi: 10.1016/j.amjcard.2012.02.019.

[52] Deedwania P, Barter P, Carmena R, Fruchart JC, et al. Treating to New Targets Investigators. Reduction of low-density lipoprotein cholesterol in patients with coronary heart disease and metabolic syndrome: analysis of the Treating to New Targets study. Lancet. 2006 Sep 9;368(9539):919-28.

[53] Arca M. Atorvastatin efficacy in the prevention of cardiovascular events in patients with diabetes mellitus and/or metabolic syndrome. Drugs. 2007;67 Suppl 1:43-54

[54] Gibson CM, Pride YB, Hochberg CP, Sloan S, Sabatine MS, Cannon CP; TIMI Study Group. Effect of intensive statin therapy on clinical outcomes among patients undergoing percutaneous coronary intervention for acute coronary syndrome. PCI-PROVE IT: A PROVE IT-TIMI 22 (Pravastatin or Atorvastatin Evaluation and Infection Therapy-Thrombolysis In Myocardial Infarction 22) Substudy. J Am Coll Cardiol. 2009; 54: 2290-22955. doi: 10.1016/j.jacc.2009.09.010.

[55] Murphy SA, Cannon CP, Wiviott SD, McCabe CH, Braunwald E. Reduction in recurrent cardiovascular events with intensive lipid-lowering statin therapy compared with moderate lipid-lowering statin therapy after acute coronary syndromes from the PROVE IT-TIMI 22 (Pravastatin or Atorvastatin Evaluation and Infection Therapy-Thrombolysis In Myocardial Infarction 22) trial. J Am Coll Cardiol. 2009; 54: 2358-2362. doi: 10.1016/j.jacc.2009.10.005.

[56] sley WL1; PROVE-IT-TIMI 22. What did PROVE-IT prove?. Diabetes Technol Ther. 2004 Dec;6(6):864-867.

[57] Pedersen TR, Cater NB, Faergeman O, Kastelein JJ, et al. Comparison of atorvastatin 80 mg/day versus simvastatin 20 to 40 mg/day on frequency of cardiovascular events late (five years) after acute myocardial infarction (from the Incremental Decrease in End Points through Aggressive Lipid Lowering [IDEAL] trial). Am J Cardiol. 2010; 106: 354-359. doi: 10.1016/j.amjcard.2010.03.033.

[58] Knopp RH, d'Emden M, Smilde JG, Pocock SJ. Efficacy and safety of atorvastatin in the prevention of cardiovascular end points in subjects with type 2 diabetes: the

Atorvastatin Study for Prevention of Coronary Heart Disease Endpoints in non-insu-lin-dependent diabetes mellitus (ASPEN). Diabetes Care. 2006; 29:1478-1485.

[59] Isaacsohn JL, Davidson MH, Hunninghake D, Singer R, McLain R, Black DM. Aggressive Lipid-Lowering Initiation Abates New Cardiac Events (ALLIANCE)-rationale and design of atorvastatin versus usual care in hypercholesterolemic patients with coronary artery disease. Am J Cardiol. 2000; 86: 250-252.

[60] Koren MJ. Statin use in a "real-world" clinical setting: aggressive lipid lowering compared with usual care in the Aggressive Lipid-Lowering Initiation Abates New Cardiac Events (ALLIANCE) trial. Am J Med. 2005; 118 Suppl 12A: 16-21.

[61] Koren MJ, Davidson MH, Wilson DJ, Fayyad RS, Zuckerman A, Reed DP; ALLIANCE Investigators. Focused atorvastatin therapy in managed-care patients with coronary heart disease and CKD. Am J Kidney Dis. 2009; 53: 741-750. doi: 10.1053/j.ajkd.2008.11.025.

[62] Mikhailidis DP, Wierzbicki AS. The GREek Atorvastatin and Coronary-heart-disease Evaluation (GREACE) study. Curr Med Res Opin. 2002; 18: 215-219.

[63] Athyros VG, Mikhailidis DP, Papageorgiou AA, Bouloukos VI, et al. Effect of statins and aspirin alone and in combination on clinical outcome in dyslipidaemic patients with coronary heart disease. A subgroup analysis of the GREACE study. Platelets. 2005; 16: 65-71.

[64] Kinlay S, Schwartz GG, Olsson AG, Rifai N, Bao W, Libby P, Ganz P; Myocardial Ischemia Reduction with Aggressive Cholesterol Lowering (MIRACL) Study Investigators. Endogenous tissue plasminogen activator and risk of recurrent cardiac events after an acute coronary syndrome in the MIRACL study. Atherosclerosis. 2009; 206: 551-555. doi: 10.1016/j.atherosclerosis.2009.03.020.

[65] Zamani P, Schwartz GG, Olsson AG, Rifai N, Bao W, Libby P, Ganz P, Kinlay S; Myocardial Ischemia Reduction with Aggressive Cholesterol Lowering (MIRACL) Study Investigators. Inflammatory biomarkers, death, and recurrent nonfatal coronary events after an acute coronary syndrome in the MIRACL study. J Am Heart Assoc. 2013; 2: e003103. doi: 10.1161/JAHA.112.003103.

[66] Arca M, Gaspardone A. Atorvastatin efficacy in the primary and secondary prevention of cardiovascular events. Drugs. 2007;67 Suppl 1:29-42.

[67] Athyros VG, Karagiannis A, Ganotakis ES, Paletas K, et al. Assessing The Treatment Effect in Metabolic syndrome without Perceptible diabetes (ATTEMPT) Collaborative Group. Curr Med Res Opin. 2011; 27: 1659-1668. doi: 10.1185/03007995.2011.595782.

[68] Plosker GL, Lyseng-Williamson KA. Atrovastatin. a pharmacoeconomic review of its use in the primary and secondary prevention of cardiovascular events. Pharmacoeconomics. 2007; 25: 1031-1053.

[69] Hawa MI, Buchan AP, Ola T, Wun CC, et al. LADA and CARDS: a prospective study of clinical outcome in established adult-onset autoimmune diabetes. Diabetes Care. 2014; 37: 1643-1649. doi: 10.2337/dc13-2383.

[70] olse H, Sternhufvud C, Andy Schuetz C, Rengarajan B, Gandhi S. Impact of switching treatment from rosuvastatin to atorvastatin on rates of cardiovascular events. Clin Ther. 2014; 36: 58-69. doi: 10.1016/j.clinthera.2013.12.003.

[71] Amarenco P, Callahan A 3rd, Campese VM, Goldstein LB, et al. Effect of High-Dose Atorvastatin on Renal Function in Subjects With Stroke or Transient Ischemic Attack in the SPARCL Trial. Stroke. 2014; 45: 2974-82. doi: 10.1161/STROKEAHA.114.005832.

[72] arma A, Cannon CP, de Lemos J, Rouleau JL, et al. The incidence of kidney injury for patients treated with a high-potency versus moderate-potency statin regimen after an acute coronary syndrome. J Am Heart Assoc. 2014; 3: e000784. doi: 10.1161/JAHA.114.000784.

[73] Mullins CD, Rattinger GB, Kuznik A, Koren MJ. Cost-effectiveness of intensive atorvastatin treatment in high-risk patients compared with usual care in a postgeneric statin market: economic analysis of the Aggressive Lipid-lowering Initiation Abates New Cardiac Events (ALLIANCE) study. Clin Ther. 2008;30 Pt 2:2204-16. doi: 10.1016/j.clinthera.2008.12.007.

[74] Annemans L, Marbaix S, Webb K, Van Gaal L, Scheen A. Cost effectiveness of atorvastatin in patients in type 2 diabetes mellitus: a pharmacoeconomic analysis of the collaborative atrovastatin diabetes study in the Belgian population. Clin Drug Investig. 2010; 30: 133-142. Doi: 10.2165/1153910-000000000-00000.

[75] Bener A, Dogan M, Barakat L, Al-Hamag AO. Comparison of cost-effectiveness, safety, and efficacy of rosuvastatin versus atrvastatin, pravastatin, and simbastatin in dyslipidemic diabetic patients with or without metabolic syndrome. J Prim Care Community Health. 2014; 11: 180-187.

[76] Parthan A, Leahy KJ, O'Sullivan AK, Iakoubova OA, et al. Cost effectiveness of targeted high-atorvastatin therapy following genotype testing in patients with acute coronary syndrome. Pharmacoeconomics. 2013; 31: 519-531. doi: 10.1007/s40273-013-0054-5.

[77] Silva MA, Swanson AC, Gandhi PJ, Tataronis GR. Statin-related adverse events: a meta-analysis. Clin Ther. 2006; 28: 26-35.

[78] Jukema JW, Cannon CP, de Craen AJ, Westendorp RG, Trompet S. The controversies of statin therapy: weighing the evidence. J Am Coll Cardiol. 2012; 40: 875-881. doi: 10.1016/j.jacc.2012.07.007.

[79] Sondermeijer BM, Boekholdt SM, Rana JS, Kastelein JJ, Wareham NJ, Khaw KT. Clinical implications of JUPITER in a contemporary European population: the EPIC-Nor-

folk prospective population study. Eur Heart J. 2013; 34: 1350-1357. doi: 10.1093/eurheartj/eht047.

[80] Teng JF, Gomes T, Camacho X, Grundy S, Juurlink DN, Mamdani MM. Impact of the JUPITER trial on statin prescribing for primary prevention. Pharmacotherapy. 2014; 34:9-18. doi: 10.1002/phar.1340.

[81] Khera AV, Everett BM, Caulfield MP, Hantash FM, Wohlgemuth J, Ridker PM, Mora S. Lipoprotein(a) concentrations, rosuvastatin therapy, and residual vascular risk: an analysis from the JUPITER Trial (Justification for the Use of Statins in Prevention: an Intervention Trial Evaluating Rosuvastatin). Circulation. 2014; 129: 635-642. doi: 10.1161/CIRCULATIONAHA.113.004406.

[82] Rajpathak SN, Kumbhani DJ, Crandall J, Brazilai N, Alderman M, Ridker PM. Statin therapy and risk of developing type 2 diabetes: a meta-analysis. Diabetes Care. 2009; 32: 1924-1929. doi: 10.2337/dc09-0738.

[83] Sampson UK, Linton MF, Fazio S. Are statins diabetogenic? Curr Opin Cardiol. 2011; 26: 342-347. doi: 10.1097/HCO.0b013e3283470359.

[84] Waters DD, Ho JE, DeMicco DA, Breazna A, Arsenault BJ, Wun CC, Kastelein JJ, Colhoun H, Barter P. Predictors of new-onset diabetes in patients treated with atorvastatin: results from 3 large randomized clinical trials. J Am Coll Cardiol. 2011; 57: 1535-1545. doi: 10.1016/j.jacc.2010.10.047

[85] Athyros VG, Elisaf MS, Alexandrides T, Achimastos A, et al. Assessing the Treatment Effect in Metabolic Syndrome Without Perceptible Diabetes (ATTEMP) Collaborative Group. Long-term impact of multifactorial treatment on new-onset diabetes and related cardiovascular events in metabolic syndrome: a post-hoc ATTEMPT analysis. Angiology. 2012; 63: 358-366. doi: 10.1177/0003319711421341.

[86] Muscoqiuri G, Sarno G, Gastaldelli A, Savastano S, Ascione A, et al. The good and bad effects of statins on insulin sensitivity and secretion. Endocr Res. 2014; 30: 137-143. doi: 10.3109/07435800.2014.952018.

[87] Simic I, Reiner Z. Adverse effects of statins-Myths and reality.Curr Pharm Des. 2014 Oct 13. [Epub ahead of print].

[88] Vidt DG, Ridker PM, Monyak JT, Schreiber MJ, Cressman MD. Longitudinal assessment of estimated glomerular filtration rate in apparently healthy adults: a posy hoc analysis from the JUPITER study (justification for the use of statins in prevention: an intervention trial evaluating rosuvastatin. Clin Ther. 2011; 33: 717-725. doi: 10.1016/.clinthera.2011.05.004.

3

Diabetic Ketoacidosis in the Pediatric Population with Type 1 Diabetes

Michal Cohen, Smadar Shilo, Nehama Zuckerman-Levin and Naim Shehadeh

Abstract

Diabetic ketoacidosis (DKA) is a leading cause of morbidity and mortality in patients with type 1 diabetes (T1DM). Individuals familiar with this complication of diabetes should be able to identify the earliest signs and symptoms and act promptly to prevent further deterioration. However, even in patients with established diabetes, the rates of DKA are considerable. This chapter discusses in detail the various aspects of DKA in the pediatric population with T1DM. The prevalence and regional effects on the prevalence of DKA as well as the specific risk factors, whether disease, patient, or physician related, are reviewed. Patients with DKA experience a condition of starvation despite the abundance of metabolic substrate (i.e., glucose); the pathophysiological mechanisms responsible for the development of DKA are outlined. Next, a detailed discussion of the clinical aspects of DKA is provided. This includes the clinical findings at presentation, the approach to treatment, and potential complications. Prevention is the best method for reducing rates of DKA. Somewhat different factors apply in patients with new-onset diabetes when compared with those with established diabetes and these are reviewed.

Keywords: Diabetic ketoacidosis, pediatrics, type 1 diabetes, epidemiology, treatment

1. Introduction

Diabetic ketoacidosis (DKA) is an acute life-threatening complication of type 1 diabetes (T1DM). Despite our detailed knowledge of this condition, rates of occurrence both in new-onset diabetes and in established diabetes are significant. This chapter will discuss various aspects of DKA in the pediatric population with T1DM, ranging from epidemiology and pathophysiology through the spectrum of clinical considerations, including the clinical presentation, diagnosis, treatment, and complications, and will end with a discussion of the importance and means for prevention of DKA.

Chapter outline:

- Epidemiology of DKA in the pediatric population
- Pathophysiology of DKA
- Clinical presentation and diagnosis of DKA
- DKA Treatment in children
- Complications of pediatric DKA
- Prevention of pediatric DKA
- Conclusion

2. Epidemiology of DKA in the pediatric population

Despite our thorough understanding of the pathophysiology of this potentially life-threatening complication of T1DM, DKA remains a relatively common occurrence in childhood diabetes.

2.1. DKA at diagnosis of T1DM

2.1.1. DKA prevalence

The prevalence of DKA at T1DM diagnosis varies greatly worldwide and ranges between 13% and 80% in different countries [1-11]. A large systematic review of 65 studies including over 29,000 children worldwide found that the lowest prevalences were reported in Sweden, Canada, the Slovak Republic, and Finland and the highest prevalences in the United Arab Emirates, Saudi Arabia, and Romania [1]. Latitude and the regional background incidence of T1DM were negatively associated with the prevalence of DKA [1, 10, 12]. Increased incidence of T1DM has previously been associated with more northern latitudes, although it is unclear whether this represents a true environmental effect or rather reflects ethnic and racial variations between populations [13, 14]. Taken together, these associations suggest that decreased awareness to T1DM and related complications may be a risk factor for DKA at diabetes diagnosis. To further support this, lack of a family history of diabetes was shown to increase the risk of presenting with DKA at diabetes diagnosis [7, 15]. However, despite the increasing incidence of T1DM around the world in recent decades [16], and therefore potentially increased awareness, the prevalence of DKA at diagnosis appears to remain stable [5, 6, 9, 17]. Data from the Search for Diabetes in Youth study (SEARCH), a multicenter US study, found that rates remained stable during 8 years of follow-up for the whole pediatric group as well as when assessing separately the younger children (<4 years of age) and the older children and [9]. They also did not detect any significant gender or ethnicity-specific changes over time.

2.1.2. Risk factors for DKA

The majority of data points to similar rates of DKA at diabetes diagnosis in boys and girls worldwide [7, 9, 11, 12, 15] (Table 1). However, one study based in Germany did suggest a slightly increased prevalence in girls [4] and another suggested increased prevalence in girls when assessing the very young age-group, under 2 years of age [3]. A younger age at diabetes diagnosis is consistently identified as an important risk factor related to DKA at presentation [2, 3, 6, 7, 9, 15, 18]. In a systematic review of 46 studies involving 24,000 children worldwide, younger age was found to be the most common factor associated with increased risk for DKA at diabetes diagnosis [12]. Different age cutoffs between 2 and 5 years of age were used in studies to describe this association. Odds ratios higher than 4 were found for Finnish children under 2 years of age when compared to those 2 years or older [19, 20]. In the SEARCH study increased prevalence of DKA at presentation was detected in children less than 4 years of age, particularly when compared to youth 15–19 years of age [7]. The causes for this increased prevalence in younger children are likely multiple. Younger children are more prone to misdiagnosis when initially presenting with T1DM [21]. This can reflect a lower index of suspicion on the physician's side combined with the difficulty of identifying the classic symptoms in a toddler; infants and young children might not be able to describe symptoms, and findings may be similar to those of other acute illnesses. However, toddlers may actually suffer a more aggressive progression of metabolic decompensation. There is evidence that younger children have a shorter prodromal period [22] as well as a more rapid decline in beta cell reserve after diabetes diagnosis [19, 23]. A lower BMI or weight loss have also been associated with increased risk for DKA at diagnosis in a number of small studies [15, 24]. Children from ethnic minorities are at increased risk for DKA at T1DM onset [12]. In the United States, higher rates of DKA at diagnosis have been recorded in Hispanic and African American youth when compared with non-Hispanic white North-American youth [9]. In the UK, children from an Asian background were at increased risk of presenting with DKA, particularly if under 5 years of age[11]. Another study from the UK demonstrated that children from non-white ethnicity were at higher risk of a delayed T1DM diagnosis and that a delayed diagnosis was associated with increased risk of DKA at presentation [25]. In the Israeli Negev, the prevalence of DKA at diabetes diagnosis was significantly higher in the Bedouin minority when compared to either the general population or the Jewish population [26]. In another study from Israel, children from an Ethiopian origin had an increased prevalence of DKA at presentation [15]. However, this is not supported by all studies, and others did not find a predilection to minority groups [7, 27]. Another predictor of DKA is a lower socioeconomic status [28]. Several components of the socioeconomic status have been identified as significant. Lower household income was found in US and Canadian studies to be a risk factor [2, 7, 9]; however, European studies did not necessarily support this [29]. In the United States, lack of private health insurance was also identified [7, 9, 30]. More years of parental education as well as academic education of the parents were found protective [7, 31, 32]. However, even in the more privileged populations, the rate of DKA at diagnosis of diabetes is substantial and recorded to occur in over 20% of patients [7]. "Physician-dependent" factors may also increase the risk for DKA at diabetes diagnosis. Such factors include delayed diagnosis of diabetes or a missed diagnosis [25, 21], delayed presentation to secondary care, or delayed treatment after T1DM diagnosis [10, 17].

Risk factors for diabetic ketoacidosis at diabetes diagnosis	
Patient specific	Younger age
	Ethnic minority
	Lower socioeconomic status
Physician related	Delayed diabetes diagnosis
	Delayed initiation of treatment
Epidemiological	Lower regional background prevalence of T1DM
	Residence in a less northern latitude
Risk factors for recurrent diabetic ketoacidosis	
	Insulin omission and poor adherence to treatment
	Poor metabolic control
	Previous episodes of DKA
	Behavioral and psychiatric disorders
	Higher levels of family conflict
	Lower socioeconomic status
	Limited access to outpatient diabetes care

Table 1. Risk factors for diabetic ketoacidosis in the pediatric population

2.2. DKA in patients with established T1DM

Recurrent DKA is by large a preventable complication in patients with established T1DM. In a large cohort of 1243 children with T1DM, the incidence of DKA in patients with established T1DM was 8/100 person-years [33]. Another study assessing a large database of children with established T1DM from Germany and Austria evaluated the incidence of DKA in the most recent year of follow-up [34]. They found that 6% of children suffered from DKA, 5% had a single episode, and 1% had two or more episodes. Two smaller studies followed children with T1DM for about 8 years and found 20–28% to experience at least one episode of DKA [26, 35]. As reflected in these data, it is estimated that it is the same small proportion of patients (around 20%) that account for the majority of admissions for DKA [33, 36]. Insulin omission and poor adherence to treatment are major risk factors [37] (Table 1). Poorer diabetes control, higher hemoglobin A1c, higher insulin doses, and previous episodes of DKA are also important risk factors [33, 34, 38]. Recurrent DKA episodes peak in teenage years, particularly in females [33, 34]. Moreover, the incidence of DKA was found to increase with age in females, yet remained stable in males. A study evaluating the role of patient and family psychosocial functioning as predictors of recurrent acute diabetic complications [35] found girls with recurrent DKA to demonstrate lower social competence and higher rates of behavioral problems. The families exhibited higher levels of family conflict and decreased family cohesion and organization. Major psychiatric disorders have also been implicated in recurrent DKA [39]. As is the case in DKA at T1DM diagnosis, lower socioeconomic status and limited access to outpatient diabetes care are also predictors of recurrent DKA [39].

3. Pathophysiology of DKA in children

By definition, hyperglycemia and ketoacidosis are the major components of DKA [40]. The initial impairment leading to DKA is an absolute or relative insulin deficiency. The sequence of events that follows leads to a patient that suffers hyperglycemia, dehydration, acidosis, electrolyte deficiencies, and variable degrees of cerebral dysfunction [41] (Figure 1). In a patient with new-onset diabetes, the cause for the insulin deficiency is the progressive deterioration in beta cell reserve and function [42]. In patients with established diabetes, insulin omission (intentional, as a result of insulin pump failure or other technical problems, or related to lack of access to medical care) is a major cause. Acute stress, commonly induced by an intercurrent illness, might precipitate DKA. During stress, counterregulatory hormone (glucagon, cortisol, growth hormone, and epinephrine) levels increase, causing hyperglycemia and an increased requirement for insulin. If this increased need for insulin is not met, DKA may ensue. Furthermore, an acute illness may impair the child's ability to replace fluid losses.

Insulin deficiency leads to hyperglycemia as a result of decreased utilization of glucose at the same time of increased hepatic and renal glucose production. Hyperglycemia increases serum osmolality, and in response, thirst is induced and osmotic diuresis occurs. The increased fluid loss further promotes polydipsia. Because of the unavailability of glucose to tissues, compensatory mechanisms are activated. Counterregulatory hormones are secreted, leading to increased glucose production by gluconeogenesis and glycogenolysis [43]. Insulin resistance increases and lipolysis is promoted, resulting in production of free fatty acids (FFAs). FFAs are metabolized into ketone bodies, particularly β-hydroxybutyrate, by the liver as an alternative energy source. The accumulation of ketones leads to metabolic acidosis. Another result of the decreased insulin and elevated counterregulatory hormone levels is proteolysis and reduced production of proteins. By this mechanism, substrates for gluconeogenesis are added, further contributing to the hyperglycemia. Initially, plasma ketone body levels rise, causing ketonemia and a base deficit; compensating mechanisms are activated and might lead to measurement of a normal pH. As the condition progresses, ketones further accumulate, ketonuria occurs, and eventually the metabolic acidosis becomes evident. The ketoacidosis causes decreased bowel motility, particularly of the small bowel, accompanied by nausea and vomiting. At this stage, the patient may be unable to compensate for the urinary fluid losses. In a vicious cycle, dehydration impairs the renal ability to clear glucose and ketoacids, thus further worsening the hyperglycemia and acidosis. The increasing osmolality, dehydration, and acidosis decrease cerebral function. This might be manifested as lethargy, or even an altered level of consciousness, further impairing the patient's ability to rehydrate. At presentation, the degree of dehydration ranges from mild to severe, with the majority of children presenting with moderate degrees of dehydration [44]. To compensate for the acidosis, respiratory mechanisms are activated, causing the labored, rapid, deep breathing typically described in patients with DKA (i.e., Kussmaul respirations). The acetone released in the breath results in a characteristic fruity odor.

Serum hyperglycemia and hyperosmolarity together with the acidosis and osmotic diuresis lead to significant electrolyte deficiencies and imbalances [40, 45, 46].

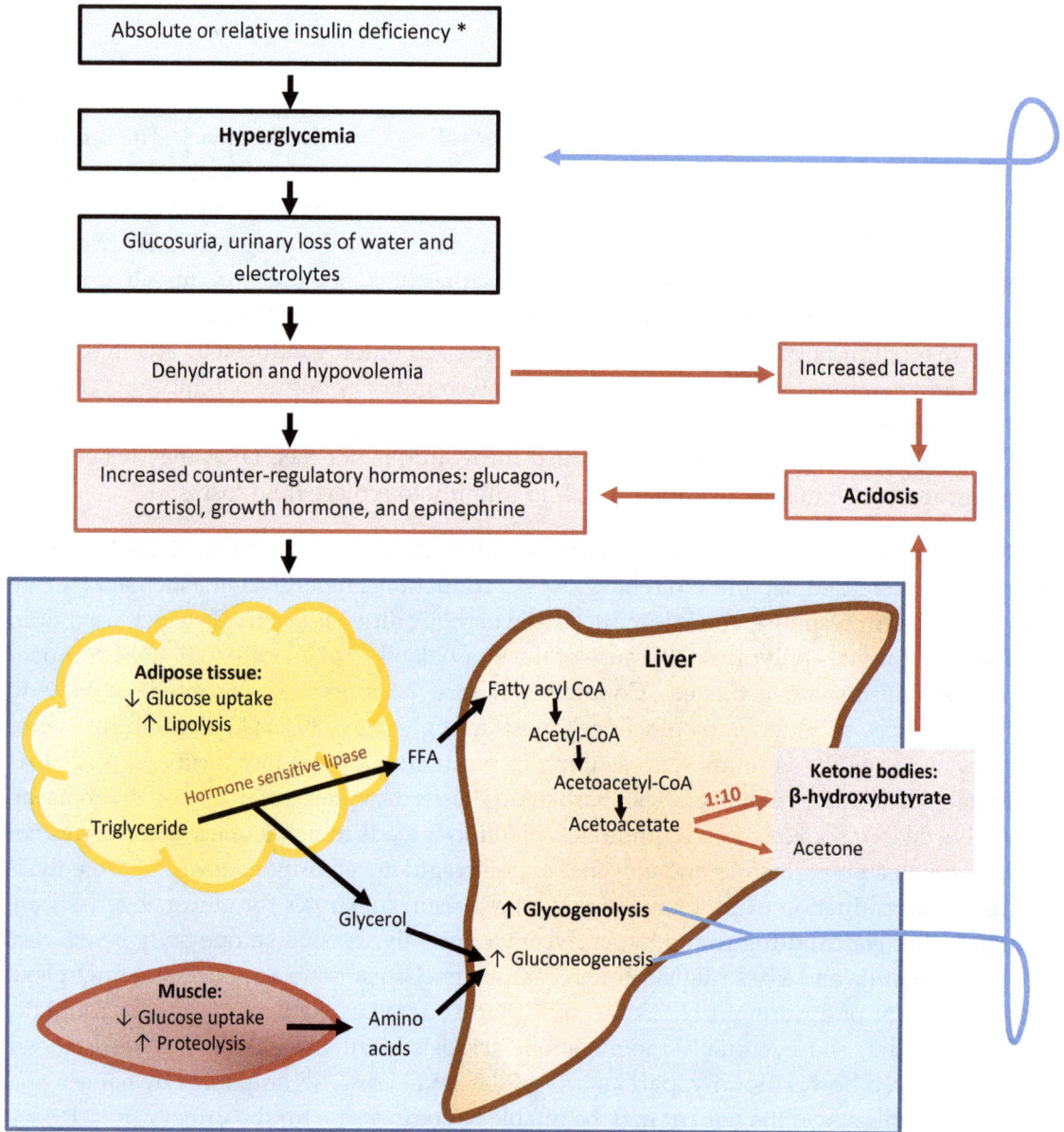

* May be induced by stress, infection, or inadequate insulin dosing in a patient with diabetes. FFA = free fatty acids.

Figure 1. Pathophysiology of diabetic ketoacidosis.

3.1. Potassium depletion

Total body stores of potassium are depleted in basically every patient with DKA, and the average potassium loss is 5 mmol/kg body weight. However, the serum potassium levels may not reflect these losses, and the actual level may be low, normal, or even elevated, particularly if renal function is impaired. The entry of hydrogen ions, accumulated extracellularly due to the acidosis, into cells drives out the intracellular potassium. The osmotic diuresis together with the high levels of aldosterone secreted as a result of the dehydration cause significant urinary loss of potassium. Emesis might cause further loss of potassium through the gastro-intestinal tract. However, an exception is patients with severe volume depletion, in whom renal insufficiency may lead to hyperkalemia. During treatment of DKA, both the insulin itself and the reversal of acidosis generate a net shift of potassium back into cells. Moreover, there is some evidence suggesting a kaliuretic effect of insulin [47]. Altogether, these may result in severe hypokalemia. Patients with hypokalemia at presentation likely suffer more severe total body potassium depletion and are at particular risk of severe hypokalemia and cardiac instability as treatment is provided.

3.2. Sodium and chloride depletion

The osmotic diuresis in DKA results in urinary loss of sodium, and the hyperosmolar state drives water out of cells into the extracellular space, leading to dilutional hyponatremia. The average sodium loss is 6 mmol/kg body weight. Chloride is secreted in the urine with sodium, and the loss is on average 4 mmol/kg body weight. It should be kept in mind that the administration of chloride during the treatment of DKA may lead to hyperchloremic metabolic acidosis, thus interfering with the correction of acidosis.

3.3. Phosphate depletion

Phosphate shifted extracellularly by the acidosis is then lost in the urine. Phosphate losses can be substantial and are estimated to be about 0.5–2.5 mmol/kg body weight. Significant hypophosphatemia has the potential to impair oxygen delivery to tissues and cause muscle weakness. However, despite very low serum levels of phosphate in some patients, such complications are rare, and studies did not demonstrate a benefit for phosphorous replacement [48, 49].

Beyond the electrolyte deficiencies described, in recent years, several studies have pointed out that a deficiency of thiamine (vitamin B1), a water-soluble vitamin of the B complex, may be clinically significant in patients with DKA. Thiamine deficiency was found to be common in children with DKA and may worsen with treatment [50]. The role of this deficiency in the clinical presentation of DKA is yet to be revealed.

4. Clinical presentation and diagnosis of DKA

Metabolic decompensation in DKA usually develops over a period of hours to a few days. Progression can be particularly rapid in patients with established diabetes. Misdiagnosis of a patient with new-onset diabetes may lead to deterioration of the metabolic status. Particularly in young children, misdiagnosis may be a result of the nonspecific symptoms and signs often described in DKA. The earliest clinical manifestations of DKA are related to hyperglycemia and may differ according to age, length of prodromal period, degree of acidosis, and volume depletion [51, 52]. Symptoms and signs in DKA are most often related to the hyperglycemia, dehydration, and acidosis [4, 53-55].

4.1. Symptoms

- Polydipsia, polyuria, and/or nocturia are almost always present, although often not reported.

- Nocturnal or daytime secondary enuresis is often described; polyphagia and weight loss may occur.

- As a result of the acidosis, patients may suffer nausea, vomiting, abdominal pain, shortness of breath, lethargy, or fatigue.

4.2. Physical signs

- Dehydration: Children with DKA often present with 5–10% fluid deficit [51, 56]. They may lack the classical signs of hypovolemia and dehydration because of the acute and chronic losses of both extracellular and intracellular water [57]. Findings depend on the degree of dehydration and may include dry oral mucosa and decreased skin turgor, tachycardia, a sunken fontanelle, and/or sunken eyes. Most patients are normotensive, although postural hypotension can occur.

- Tachypnea or Kussmaul (deep, sighing, and labored) respiration with a fruity acetone odor.

- Signs of decreased tissue perfusion such as a slow capillary refill.

- Neurologic findings [58]: from confusion and drowsiness to decreased consciousness and coma. Neurologic findings should raise the suspicion of cerebral edema.

In infants, especially those who are not toilet trained, the diagnosis may be delayed. Weight loss, irritability, and decreased activity are common at presentation. Dehydration and severe diaper rash may be the only physical signs. Older children and adolescents can manifest profound wasting, cachexia, and prostration on DKA presentation, especially with a prolonged course of uncontrolled/misdiagnosed diabetes.

4.3. Laboratory findings

4.3.1. Diagnostic criteria

Biochemical criteria for the diagnosis of DKA are defined as follows [40, 51, 56, 59]:

- Hyperglycemia: blood glucose (BG) >200 mg/dl (11 mmol/L)

- Metabolic acidosis: venous pH <7.3 and/or bicarbonate <15 mmol/L

- Ketonemia and ketonuria: serum beta hydroxybutyrate ≥3 mmol/L

On certain occasions, patients may present with "euglycemic ketoacidosis" where glucose levels are near normal [54, 59]. This may develop in young children who consumed small amounts of carbohydrates or are partially treated or in children with emesis.

The severity of DKA is established by the degree of acidosis: mild DKA, pH 7.2–7.3 or bicarbonate <15 mmol/L; moderate DKA, pH 7.1–7.2 or bicarbonate 5–10 mmol/L; and severe

DKA, pH <7.1 or bicarbonate <5 mmol/L [51, 56, 58]. The duration of symptoms, volume deficit, degree of ketosis, and neurologic status further determine the severity of illness in a child with DKA.

4.3.2. Acid–base balance

Acidosis is caused by the production and accumulation of ketones in the serum [49]. Three ketones are produced in DKA: two ketoacids (beta-hydroxybutyrate and acetoacetate) and the neutral ketone, acetone. In DKA, beta-hydroxybutyrate constitutes 75% of the circulating ketones. During recovery, it is converted to acetoacetate and acetone, which persists for a longer period. Therefore, measuring serum beta-hydroxybutyrate is the most useful for diagnosis. The severity of the metabolic acidosis is dependent on the compensatory respiratory alkalosis, the acid excretion in the urine [60], and the duration and rate of increased ketoacid production. The serum anion gap (AG) is an index of unmeasured anions in the blood (normal in children is 12 ± 2 mEq/L). Most patients with DKA present with a high AG ($\geq$20 mEq/L) due to high serum levels of ketoacids. The resolution of ketoacidosis is followed by a normal AG.

4.3.3. Electrolyte imbalances

Laboratory tests that should be routinely monitored in the setting of DKA include serum glucose, electrolytes, creatinine and BUN, blood gases, pH, bicarbonate, and a complete blood count. Changes over time in electrolytes and renal function tests must be followed.

Serum potassium: As mentioned earlier, potassium loss can be a result of increased ketoacid excretion, osmotic diuresis, vomiting, or diarrhea. The serum potassium concentration may be normal, increased, or decreased at diagnosis of DKA. However, monitoring of potassium levels is crucial because hypokalemia may eventually develop.

Serum sodium: Low serum sodium in DKA may occur due to hyperglycemia and its effect on plasma osmolarity. Polydipsia and excessive consumption of water can also contribute to lowering sodium concentration. Osmotic dieresis and water loss in excess of sodium and potassium will tend to raise the serum sodium concentration. Hyperlipidemia can cause pseudohyponatremia [61].

Serum phosphate: Decreased phosphate intake and phosphaturia may result in a negative phosphate balance. At presentation of DKA, serum phosphate is usually normal or high due to the combined effect of metabolic acidosis and insulin deficiency. The degree of phosphate loss in DKA is apparent after insulin treatment [62].

4.4. Differential diagnosis of DKA

DKA should be differentiated from other causes of acidosis and/or hyperglycemia, such as acute gastroenteritis with metabolic acidosis, uremia, salicylate intoxication, starvation ketosis and lactic acidosis. When the presenting symptom is altered consciousness or coma, encephalitis and other CNS pathologies must be ruled out. Diabetic ketoacidosis should also be distinguished from the hyperosmolar hyperglycemic state, which is infrequent in children [51, 57, 63]. The main differences between these conditions are the degree of acidosis and insulinopenia.

5. DKA treatment in children

Successful treatment of DKA requires correction of dehydration, acid–base and electrolyte imbalances, insulin administration, and identification of comorbid and precipitating conditions. This treatment may be associated with inherent risks of inducing hypoglycemia, hypokalemia, and cerebral edema. Therefore, any protocol must be used with caution, and close monitoring of patients is crucial. Children with severe DKA, an altered level of consciousness, or those who are at increased risk for complications should be considered for treatment in an intensive care setting. In this chapter, we will focus on the general principals and considerations in DKA management as well as controversies regarding DKA treatment.

5.1. Standard protocols for DKA management

There is some variability in protocols for DKA management, but the basic principles are similar in the various protocols available in the literature [40, 51, 64, 65]. Protocols enabling standardization of treatment are of great value to the treating team involved; however, clinical judgment should always be practiced. Frequent monitoring of the patient is a very important aspect of the treatment and should include meticulous documentation of clinical observations, fluid balance, laboratory results, and medications administered. A neurological follow-up for warning signs and symptoms of cerebral edema is also essential.

5.2. Fluid replacement

Fluid replacement in children with DKA remains a controversial topic with regard to the amount of intravenous fluid, rate of delivery, and fluid composition. Current recommendations are based on expert consensus statements and accumulated clinical experience, as evidence from large randomized clinical trials is lacking.

5.2.1. First hour fluid resuscitation

The goals of initial volume expansion are to restore the effective circulating volume and the glomerular filtration rate. Intravenous fluid administration bares the risk of inducing an elevation in the intracranial pressure (ICP), potentially resulting in cerebral edema, and thus should be done carefully [66, 67]. In a rabbit model of DKA, the use of hypotonic fluids, compared with isotonic, was associated with greater rises in ICP [66]. Some studies suggest that rapid fluid replacement may increase the risk of cerebral edema [68, 69], although other studies did not support this finding [70, 71]. Studies in both adults and children demonstrated a more rapid correction of acidosis when a slower rate of fluid administration with isotonic or near-isotonic solutions was used [72, 73]. Hyperchloremic metabolic acidosis is another often overlooked risk resulting from the use of large volumes of normal saline (NS) (0.9%) [73, 74]. At present, there is no data that support the use of colloid in preference to crystalloid in the treatment of DKA. Based on these data, most protocols recommend an initial IV infusion of 10–20 ml/kg of normal saline (NS) (0.9%) or Ringer's lactate over the first 1 to 2 h of treatment. Fluid boluses may be repeated according to the patient's hemodynamic status. However, total IV fluids should not exceed 40 ml/kg in the initial 4 h of treatment due to the aforementioned risks.

5.2.2. Fluid replacement over the next 24–48 h of treatment

Once the child is hemodynamically stable, subsequent volume expansion should be given more gradually, with a goal of replacing the remaining fluid deficit over the next 24 to 72 h. Significant additional fluid loss after initiation of treatment is rare because vomiting and excessive urine output usually resolve within the first hours of treatment. Half NS or NS (0.45–0.9%) solutions are appropriate for replacement. The rate of fluid administration is guided by the estimated degree of dehydration and fluid deficit. Calculating the effective osmolality is also of use, and most often, replacement is in the range of 1.5–2 times the usual maintenance requirement based on age and weight. Unless a contraindication exists, potassium must be added at this time (see below). To prevent a rapid decrease in plasma glucose concentration and hypoglycemia, 5% glucose should be added to the IV fluid when the plasma glucose falls to approximately 250–300 mg/dl (14–17 mmol/L), or sooner if rapidly decreasing. Fluids that were given in another facility before assessment should be factored into calculation of deficit and be subtracted from the 24-h totals.

5.3. Insulin administration

5.3.1. Intravenous insulin administration

Insulin therapy is essential to suppress lipolysis and ketogenesis and to correct acidosis. Insulin infusion is recommended 1–2 h after starting fluid replacement therapy and initial volume expansion. An initial IV bolus of insulin is unnecessary, it was not shown to affect the duration of time to attaining a serum glucose level of less than 250 mg/dl, yet it may increase the risk of cerebral edema [69, 75, 76]. A slow infusion of a low dose of 0.1 U/kg/h IV insulin is considered the standard of care in pediatric DKA [77, 78]. The dose of insulin should remain 0.1 U/kg/h at least until the resolution of DKA (pH >7.30; bicarbonate >15 mmol/L and/or closure of the anion gap). It is possible that even a lower dose of insulin is sufficient for DKA treatment. A recent randomized control trial compared a very low dose IV insulin infusion (0.05 U/kg/hr) to the standard dose. Similar results were achieved in terms of the rate of blood glucose decrease and the resolution of acidosis, suggesting that a dose lower than the current standard dose can be used [78].

5.3.2. Subcutaneous insulin regimens

Few studies, mostly in adults, demonstrated subcutaneous rapid acting insulin injected every 1–2 h to be a valid alternative for the standard intravenous insulin treatment of mild-to-moderate uncomplicated DKA [79, 80]. In our practice, we administer subcutaneous regular insulin (SCRI) every 4 h for treating children with DKA and pH ≥7.00 and K >2.5 mEq/L. Insulin therapy is initiated during the second hour of treatment and administered every 4 h until resolution of DKA. The insulin dose is calculated as 0.8–1 IU/kg/day divided by 6. This treatment was found to be a simple, effective, and safe alternative to the standard DKA protocol. Such treatment has the potential to simplify insulin administration and reduce both patient inconvenience and admission costs. Subcutaneous insulin should not be used in subjects whose peripheral circulation is impaired.

5.4. Electrolyte replacements

5.4.1. Potassium replacement

Children with DKA suffer from total body potassium deficits of approximately 3–6 mmol/kg. Hypokalemia at presentation may be related to prolonged duration of disease, whereas hyperkalemia primarily results from reduced renal function [60]. Insulin administration and the correction of acidosis drive potassium back into the cells, which may cause hypokalemia and predispose the patient to cardiac arrhythmias. Replacement therapy is usually required regardless of the serum potassium concentration. In most protocols, potassium is not given during the first hour of fluid resuscitation unless the patient is hypokalemic, in which case some protocols recommend adding potassium to the initial volume expansion before starting insulin therapy. Potassium can be given as potassium phosphate or potassium chloride. The starting potassium concentration in the infusate should be 40 mmol/L. Subsequent potassium therapy should be based on serum potassium measurements.

5.4.2. Phosphate and calcium replacement

Prospective studies have not shown clinical benefit from phosphate replacement [48, 49, 81]. The deficit usually corrects spontaneously, although it should be kept in mind that it may persist for several days after the resolution of DKA [45]. Therefore, only severe and symptomatic hypophosphatemia accompanied by significant weakness should be treated with phosphate supplements. Potassium phosphate may be used safely in combination with potassium chloride or acetate to avoid hyperchloremia. Careful monitoring of serum calcium should be performed to avoid hypocalcemia. In a study on nine children with DKA, during phosphate infusion, transient hypocalcemia occurred in 67% and transient hypomagnesemia in 56%. One child developed carpopedal spasms refractory to intravenous infusion of calcium gluconate but responsive to intramuscular injection of magnesium sulfate. In 33%, parathyroid hormone was low at the time of hypocalcemia, an observation that suggests transient hypoparathyroidism [82].

5.4.3. Bicarbonate therapy

Acidosis is reversible by insulin replacement. Several clinical trials have shown no clinical benefit from bicarbonate administration in pediatric DKA [83-86]. Moreover, bicarbonate therapy may cause paradoxical CNS acidosis. Bicarbonate crosses the blood–brain barrier slowly, yet the CO_2 formed ($HCO_3 + H+ \rightarrow H_2O + CO_2$) crosses rapidly into the CNS forming

H_2CO_3, thus worsening the CNS acidosis [87, 88]. As a result of the sodium supplement included in the bicarbonate preparations, this therapy may be associated with hypokalemia and increasing osmolality. Bicarbonate administration was also reported as a risk factor for cerebral edema in several studies [51, 69, 89]. Despite all the risks mentioned, in must be kept in mind that patients with severe acidemia (arterial pH ≤6.9) in whom decreased cardiac contractility and peripheral vasodilatation can further impair tissue perfusion and patients with life-threatening hyperkalemia may benefit from cautious alkali therapy [84]. If bicarbonate is considered necessary, it should be cautiously administered at a dose of 1–2 mmol/kg over 60 min.

5.5. Introduction of oral fluids and transition to SC insulin injections

Upon resolution of DKA and when substantial clinical improvement has occurred, oral fluids can be introduced and a protocol of subcutaneous insulin can be initiated or restarted.

6. Complications of pediatric DKA

As mentioned in detail earlier, diabetic ketoacidosis (DKA) is treated with fluids, electrolytes, and insulin. With prompt treatment, complications of DKA are uncommon. However, when complications do occur, they are usually serious with significant mortality and long-term morbidity. Surprisingly, the most common complication of DKA (cerebral edema) may be related to this lifesaving treatment.

6.1. Cerebral edema

Cerebral edema is a devastating and unpredictable complication of DKA and its treatment. Epidemiological studies demonstrate that overall cerebral edema occurs in around 7/1000 episodes of DKA and is more common in children and newly diagnosed patients. Other studies found that clinically apparent cerebral edema develops in 1–2% of children with DKA [90]. The pathophysiology of cerebral edema is not well understood, and it is likely that several processes contribute to the development of this complication: ischemic, osmotic, and vasogenic.

Osmotic: ultimately, cerebral edema is due to excessive entry of water into the cells of the central nervous system due to the presence of intracellular idiogenic osmoles causing swelling of the brain as serum osmolality drops during treatment.

Vasogenic: studies using magnetic resonance diffusion weighted imaging demonstrate that the apparent diffusion coefficient of brain water is greater during treatment of DKA than during recovery, indicating increased extracellular fluid due to an increase in blood brain barrier permeability during the acute treatment phase of DKA [91-93]. These findings are consistent with the vasogenic cerebral edema, i.e., fluid surrounding the cells, rather than osmotic cell swelling that has previously been suggested. This vasogenic theory is also supported by the fact that the degrees of dehydration and hyperventilation at presentation, but not initial osmolality or osmotic changes during treatment, were correlated with degree of edema formation [92]. This edema (within the enclosed space of the cranium) can cause transtentorial brain herniation through the foramen magnum, leading to unconsciousness and respiratory arrest.

6.1.1. Risk factors for cerebral edema

Several case–control studies have pointed out risk factors for the development of cerebral edema [69, 70, 94, 95]. These can be divided into two main groups.

Risk factors related to disease severity at presentation:

a. Younger age

b. Newly diagnosed compared with established diabetes

c. More severe acidosis at presentation

d. Higher serum urea levels

e. Lower partial arterial CO_2 ($PaCO_2$) values

Risk factors related to therapy:

a. Larger volume of fluid given during the first 4 h of treatment

b. Administration of bicarbonate

c. Lower plasma sodium concentrations

d. Administration of insulin within the first hour of treatment

6.1.2. Symptoms and signs

These typically appear within 6–24 h after starting intravenous fluids and insulin treatment. Therefore, it is crucial to monitor and recognize the early warning signs of cerebral edema through careful monitoring of all DKA patients. These include signs and symptoms of increasing intracranial pressure, such as a decline in the level of consciousness, headaches, bradycardia, depressed respiration and apnea, papillary changes, papilledema, posturing, seizures, and coma.

6.1.3. Diagnosis

The diagnosis of cerebral edema is clinical. Recognition of the above-mentioned signs and symptoms should allow early intervention and hopefully prevention of morbidities associated with this condition. CT or MRI of the brain should be performed to rule out other diagnoses and potentially confirm the diagnosis of cerebral edema. However, it should be emphasized that radiographic imaging may be unhelpful in detecting cerebral edema if performed very early after the development of symptoms.

6.1.4. Treatment of cerebral edema

The patient should be treated and monitored in the intensive care unit; however, if located elsewhere, initial treatment must not be delayed until transitioned. Mannitol or hypertonic saline should be readily available for use at the earliest signs and symptoms of cerebral edema. Other measures include a reduction in the rate of fluid administration and elevation of the head of the bed. Mannitol 1 g/kg (5 ml/kg of mannitol 20%) should be administered over 15 min; alternatively, hypertonic saline (3% NaCl) 5–10 ml/kg over 30 min can be administered. This treatment will reduce brain edema and blood viscosity and improve cerebral blood flow. Intubation and ventilation may be necessary to provide adequate ventilation and correct acidosis. Aggressive hyperventilation has been associated with poor neurological outcome and is not recommended [96].

6.2. Hypoglycemia and hypokalemia

These are additional potential complications of DKA treatment. Both are discussed earlier in the chapter.

6.3. Rare complications of DKA

6.3.1. Adult respiratory distress syndrome

This has been reported in patients with DKA, especially in patients younger than 50 years. Clinical features include dyspnea and tachypnea, with central cyanosis and nonspecific chest symptoms.

6.3.2. Acute renal failure

This can develop due to severe dehydration. Once fluid replacement is restored, kidney function should start to recover.

6.3.3. Thromboembolic complications

These may arise as a consequence of dehydration, increased blood viscosity, and coagulability. Rehydration and restoration of body fluids might help in preventing these complications [97]. Established thromboembolic complication should be treated promptly.

7. Prevention of pediatric DKA

The best approach for decreasing the burden of DKA is prevention. Preventive measures are based on the identified risk factors of T1DM and DKA and on their clinical presentation. Risk factors differ between DKA at the time of T1DM diagnosis and episodes occurring in patients with established diabetes. Identifying high-risk children, using both immunologic and genetic methods, can lead to earlier diagnosis of diabetes and decreased DKA incidence at disease onset [10, 33, 98, 99]. However, such screening raises obvious ethical questions, as the exact risk or timing of the development of diabetes in a child at risk are not known and no treatment has proved protective thus far. In families with T1DM, a special attention to early symptoms and signs is recommended to detect the onset of diabetes in other members and to prevent future DKA [51].

Greater public awareness to signs and symptoms of DKA has been related to decreased rates of DKA. This is further emphasized by the success of awareness campaigns in decreasing the rates of DKA. A campaign to increase awareness of physicians, schools, and parents was carried out in Parma, Italy [1991–1997] [100, 101]. The researchers displayed posters in pediatric centers, schools, and physician offices and demonstrated a significant reduction in the DKA rate from 78% to 12% in 6–14 years old children over an 8-year period. An Australian study demonstrated a reduction in DKA prevalence in new-onset diabetes from 38% to 14%, when repeating the Parma study diabetes awareness campaign [102]. However, it is important to mention that not all such programs have been successful [5], and complex risk factors might be involved.

The rates of DKA in patients with established diabetes can also be reduced. Identifying the specific causes for recurrent DKA in a child is important and may prevent future DKA events [40]. Detailed and intensive diabetes education programs, telephone help lines, and availability of skilled health care providers can reduce DKA occurrence [103-106]. Education programs lead to better understanding of the disease and might assist families in identifying times of increased risk (i.e., intercurrent illness or pump malfunction) as well as early signs of deterioration and of DKA. Such programs are important to the noncompliant children, especially those with recurrent episodes of DKA, and should be led by professional teams [17, 107]. Education and adult guidance were shown to decrease insulin omission in patients with recurrent DKA episodes [108]. Early identification of ketosis, using home measurement of beta-hydroxybutyrate, can prevent progression to DKA [109].

8. Conclusion

DKA is a serious complication of pediatric T1DM. The pathophysiology is complex, demonstrating reciprocal effects between the metabolic derangements involved. A "hunger" response takes place despite the abundance of metabolic substrate. Various risk factors have been identified, some are patient related yet others emphasize the important effects of both family and social circumstances. DKA is largely preventable, and efforts to further increase awareness to this complication of diabetes should be encouraged.

Author details

Michal Cohen[1*], Smadar Shilo[1], Nehama Zuckerman-Levin[1,2] and Naim Shehadeh[1,2]

*Address all correspondence to: cohenm4@gmail.com

1 Pediatric Diabetes Clinic and Pediatrics A Division, the Ruth Rappaport Children's Hospital, Rambam healthcare campus, Haifa, Israel

2 Rappaport Faculty of Medicine, Technion, Haifa, Israel

References

[1] Usher-Smith JA, Thompson M, Ercole A, Walter FM. Variation between countries in the frequency of diabetic ketoacidosis at first presentation of type 1 diabetes in children: a systematic review. Diabetologia. 2012;55(11):2878-94. Epub 2012/08/31.

[2] Bui H, To T, Stein R, Fung K, Daneman D. Is diabetic ketoacidosis at disease onset a result of missed diagnosis? The Journal of pediatrics. 2010;156(3):472-7. Epub 2009/12/08.

[3] Schober E, Rami B, Waldhoer T, Austrian Diabetes Incidence Study G. Diabetic ketoacidosis at diagnosis in Austrian children in 1989-2008: a population-based analysis. Diabetologia. 2010;53(6):1057-61. Epub 2010/03/10.

[4] Neu A, Willasch A, Ehehalt S, Hub R, Ranke MB, Baden-Wuerttemberg DG. Ketoacidosis at onset of type 1 diabetes mellitus in children--frequency and clinical presentation. Pediatric diabetes. 2003;4(2):77-81. Epub 2003/12/06.

[5] Fritsch M, Schober E, Rami-Merhar B, Hofer S, Frohlich-Reiterer E, Waldhoer T, et al. Diabetic ketoacidosis at diagnosis in Austrian children: a population-based analysis, 1989-2011. The Journal of pediatrics. 2013;163(5):1484-8 e1. Epub 2013/08/21.

[6] Lansdown AJ, Barton J, Warner J, Williams D, Gregory JW, Harvey JN, et al. Prevalence of ketoacidosis at diagnosis of childhood onset Type 1 diabetes in Wales from 1991 to 2009 and effect of a publicity campaign. Diabetic medicine : a journal of the British Diabetic Association. 2012;29(12):1506-9. Epub 2012/03/15.

[7] Rewers A, Klingensmith G, Davis C, Petitti DB, Pihoker C, Rodriguez B, et al. Presence of diabetic ketoacidosis at diagnosis of diabetes mellitus in youth: the Search for Diabetes in Youth Study. Pediatrics. 2008;121(5):e1258-66. Epub 2008/05/03.

[8] Kamal Alanani NM, Alsulaimani AA. Epidemiological pattern of newly diagnosed children with type 1 diabetes mellitus, Taif, Saudi Arabia. TheScientificWorldJournal. 2013;2013:421569. Epub 2013/11/14.

[9] Dabelea D, Rewers A, Stafford JM, Standiford DA, Lawrence JM, Saydah S, et al. Trends in the prevalence of ketoacidosis at diabetes diagnosis: the SEARCH for diabetes in youth study. Pediatrics. 2014;133(4):e938-45. Epub 2014/04/02.

[10] Levy-Marchal C, Patterson CC, Green A, Europe EASG, Diabetes. Geographical variation of presentation at diagnosis of type I diabetes in children: the EURODIAB study. European and Dibetes. Diabetologia. 2001;44 Suppl 3:B75-80. Epub 2001/11/29.

[11] Alvi NS, Davies P, Kirk JM, Shaw NJ. Diabetic ketoacidosis in Asian children. Archives of disease in childhood. 2001;85(1):60-1. Epub 2001/06/23.

[12] Usher-Smith JA, Thompson MJ, Sharp SJ, Walter FM. Factors associated with the presence of diabetic ketoacidosis at diagnosis of diabetes in children and young adults: a systematic review. Bmj. 2011;343:d4092. Epub 2011/07/09.

[13] Karvonen M, Tuomilehto J, Libman I, LaPorte R. A review of the recent epidemiological data on the worldwide incidence of type 1 (insulin-dependent) diabetes mellitus.

World Health Organization DIAMOND Project Group. Diabetologia. 1993;36(10): 883-92. Epub 1993/10/01.

[14] Karvonen M, Viik-Kajander M, Moltchanova E, Libman I, LaPorte R, Tuomilehto J. Incidence of childhood type 1 diabetes worldwide. Diabetes Mondiale (DiaMond) Project Group. Diabetes care. 2000;23(10):1516-26. Epub 2000/10/07.

[15] de Vries L, Oren L, Lazar L, Lebenthal Y, Shalitin S, Phillip M. Factors associated with diabetic ketoacidosis at onset of Type 1 diabetes in children and adolescents. Diabetic medicine : a journal of the British Diabetic Association. 2013;30(11):1360-6. Epub 2013/06/14.

[16] Group DP. Incidence and trends of childhood Type 1 diabetes worldwide 1990-1999. Diabetic medicine : a journal of the British Diabetic Association. 2006;23(8):857-66. Epub 2006/08/17.

[17] Lokulo-Sodipe K, Moon RJ, Edge JA, Davies JH. Identifying targets to reduce the incidence of diabetic ketoacidosis at diagnosis of type 1 diabetes in the UK. Archives of disease in childhood. 2014;99(5):438-42. Epub 2014/01/08.

[18] Savoldelli RD, Farhat SC, Manna TD. Alternative management of diabetic ketoacidosis in a Brazilian pediatric emergency department. Diabetology & metabolic syndrome. 2010;2:41. Epub 2010/06/17.

[19] Komulainen J, Kulmala P, Savola K, Lounamaa R, Ilonen J, Reijonen H, et al. Clinical, autoimmune, and genetic characteristics of very young children with type 1 diabetes. Childhood Diabetes in Finland (DiMe) Study Group. Diabetes care. 1999;22(12): 1950-5. Epub 1999/12/10.

[20] Hekkala A, Knip M, Veijola R. Ketoacidosis at diagnosis of type 1 diabetes in children in northern Finland: temporal changes over 20 years. Diabetes care. 2007;30(4): 861-6. Epub 2007/03/30.

[21] Mallare JT, Cordice CC, Ryan BA, Carey DE, Kreitzer PM, Frank GR. Identifying risk factors for the development of diabetic ketoacidosis in new onset type 1 diabetes mellitus. Clinical pediatrics. 2003;42(7):591-7. Epub 2003/10/14.

[22] Neu A, Ehehalt S, Willasch A, Kehrer M, Hub R, Ranke MB. Varying clinical presentations at onset of type 1 diabetes mellitus in children--epidemiological evidence for different subtypes of the disease? Pediatric diabetes. 2001;2(4):147-53. Epub 2004/03/16.

[23] Sochett EB, Daneman D, Clarson C, Ehrlich RM. Factors affecting and patterns of residual insulin secretion during the first year of type 1 (insulin-dependent) diabetes mellitus in children. Diabetologia. 1987;30(7):453-9. Epub 1987/07/01.

[24] Hekkala A, Reunanen A, Koski M, Knip M, Veijola R, Finnish Pediatric Diabetes R. Age-related differences in the frequency of ketoacidosis at diagnosis of type 1 diabetes in children and adolescents. Diabetes care. 2010;33(7):1500-2. Epub 2010/04/24.

[25] Sundaram PC, Day E, Kirk JM. Delayed diagnosis in type 1 diabetes mellitus. Archives of disease in childhood. 2009;94(2):151-2. Epub 2008/06/20.

[26] Hilmi A, Pasternak Y, Friger M, Loewenthal N, Haim A, Hershkovitz E. Ethnic differences in glycemic control and diabetic ketoacidosis rate among children with diabetes mellitus type 1 in the Negev area. The Israel Medical Association journal : IMAJ. 2013;15(6):267-70. Epub 2013/07/26.

[27] Abdul-Rasoul M, Al-Mahdi M, Al-Qattan H, Al-Tarkait N, Alkhouly M, Al-Safi R, et al. Ketoacidosis at presentation of type 1 diabetes in children in Kuwait: frequency and clinical characteristics. Pediatric diabetes. 2010;11(5):351-6. Epub 2009/10/14.

[28] Blanc N, Lucidarme N, Tubiana-Rufi N. [Factors associated with childhood diabetes manifesting as ketoacidosis and its severity]. Archives de pediatrie : organe officiel de la Societe francaise de pediatrie. 2003;10(4):320-5. Epub 2003/06/24. Facteurs associes a l'acidocetose revelatrice du diabete de l'enfant et a sa severite.

[29] Komulainen J, Lounamaa R, Knip M, Kaprio EA, Akerblom HK. Ketoacidosis at the diagnosis of type 1 (insulin dependent) diabetes mellitus is related to poor residual beta cell function. Childhood Diabetes in Finland Study Group. Archives of disease in childhood. 1996;75(5):410-5. Epub 1996/11/01.

[30] Maniatis AK, Goehrig SH, Gao D, Rewers A, Walravens P, Klingensmith GJ. Increased incidence and severity of diabetic ketoacidosis among uninsured children with newly diagnosed type 1 diabetes mellitus. Pediatric diabetes. 2005;6(2):79-83. Epub 2005/06/21.

[31] Rosenbauer J, Icks A, Giani G. Clinical characteristics and predictors of severe ketoacidosis at onset of type 1 diabetes mellitus in children in a North Rhine-Westphalian region, Germany. Journal of pediatric endocrinology & metabolism : JPEM. 2002;15(8):1137-45. Epub 2002/10/22.

[32] Sadauskaite-Kuehne V, Samuelsson U, Jasinskiene E, Padaiga Z, Urbonaite B, Edenvall H, et al. Severity at onset of childhood type 1 diabetes in countries with high and low incidence of the condition. Diabetes research and clinical practice. 2002;55(3): 247-54. Epub 2002/02/19.

[33] Rewers A, Chase HP, Mackenzie T, Walravens P, Roback M, Rewers M, et al. Predictors of acute complications in children with type 1 diabetes. Jama. 2002;287(19): 2511-8. Epub 2002/05/22.

[34] Fritsch M, Rosenbauer J, Schober E, Neu A, Placzek K, Holl RW, et al. Predictors of diabetic ketoacidosis in children and adolescents with type 1 diabetes. Experience from a large multicentre database. Pediatric diabetes. 2011;12(4 Pt 1):307-12. Epub 2011/04/07.

[35] Dumont RH, Jacobson AM, Cole C, Hauser ST, Wolfsdorf JI, Willett JB, et al. Psycho-social predictors of acute complications of diabetes in youth. Diabetic medicine : a journal of the British Diabetic Association. 1995;12(7):612-8. Epub 1995/07/01.

[36] Skinner TC. Recurrent diabetic ketoacidosis: causes, prevention and management. Hormone research. 2002;57 Suppl 1:78-80. Epub 2002/04/30.

[37] Morris AD, Boyle DI, McMahon AD, Greene SA, MacDonald TM, Newton RW. Adherence to insulin treatment, glycaemic control, and ketoacidosis in insulin-dependent diabetes mellitus. The DARTS/MEMO Collaboration. Diabetes Audit and Research in Tayside Scotland. Medicines Monitoring Unit. Lancet. 1997;350(9090): 1505-10. Epub 1997/12/06.

[38] Levine BS, Anderson BJ, Butler DA, Antisdel JE, Brackett J, Laffel LM. Predictors of glycemic control and short-term adverse outcomes in youth with type 1 diabetes. The Journal of pediatrics. 2001;139(2):197-203. Epub 2001/08/07.

[39] Rewers M. Challenges in diagnosing type 1 diabetes in different populations. Diabetes & metabolism journal. 2012;36(2):90-7. Epub 2012/04/28.

[40] Wolfsdorf J, Craig ME, Daneman D, Dunger D, Edge J, Lee W, et al. Diabetic ketoacidosis in children and adolescents with diabetes. Pediatric diabetes. 2009;10 Suppl 12:118-33. Epub 2009/09/17.

[41] Foster DW, McGarry JD. The metabolic derangements and treatment of diabetic ketoacidosis. The New England journal of medicine. 1983;309(3):159-69. Epub 1983/07/21.

[42] Matveyenko AV, Butler PC. Relationship between beta-cell mass and diabetes onset. Diabetes, obesity & metabolism. 2008;10 Suppl 4:23-31. Epub 2008/10/18.

[43] Umpierrez GE, DiGirolamo M, Tuvlin JA, Isaacs SD, Bhoola SM, Kokko JP. Differences in metabolic and hormonal milieu in diabetic- and alcohol-induced ketoacidosis. Journal of critical care. 2000;15(2):52-9. Epub 2000/07/06.

[44] Fagan MJ, Avner J, Khine H. Initial fluid resuscitation for patients with diabetic ketoacidosis: how dry are they? Clinical pediatrics. 2008;47(9):851-5. Epub 2008/07/16.

[45] Atchley DW, Loeb RF, Richards DW, Benedict EM, Driscoll ME. ON DIABETIC ACIDOSIS: A Detailed Study of Electrolyte Balances Following the Withdrawal and Reestablishment of Insulin Therapy. The Journal of clinical investigation. 1933;12(2): 297-326. Epub 1933/03/01.

[46] Nabarro JD, Spencer AG, Stowers JM. Treatment of diabetic ketosis. Lancet. 1952;1(6716):983-9. Epub 1952/05/17.

[47] Carlotti AP, St George-Hyslop C, Bohn D, Halperin ML. Hypokalemia during treatment of diabetic ketoacidosis: clinical evidence for an aldosterone-like action of insulin. The Journal of pediatrics. 2013;163(1):207-12 e1. Epub 2013/02/16.

[48] Fisher JN, Kitabchi AE. A randomized study of phosphate therapy in the treatment of diabetic ketoacidosis. The Journal of clinical endocrinology and metabolism. 1983;57(1):177-80. Epub 1983/07/01.

[49] Wilson HK, Keuer SP, Lea AS, Boyd AE, 3rd, Eknoyan G. Phosphate therapy in diabetic ketoacidosis. Archives of internal medicine. 1982;142(3):517-20. Epub 1982/03/01.

[50] Rosner EA, Strezlecki KD, Clark JA, Lieh-Lai M. Low Thiamine Levels in Children With Type 1 Diabetes and Diabetic Ketoacidosis: A Pilot Study. Pediatric critical care medicine : a journal of the Society of Critical Care Medicine and the World Federation of Pediatric Intensive and Critical Care Societies. 2014. Epub 2015/01/07.

[51] Dunger DB, Sperling MA, Acerini CL, Bohn DJ, Daneman D, Danne TP, et al. ESPE/LWPES consensus statement on diabetic ketoacidosis in children and adolescents. Archives of disease in childhood. 2004;89(2):188-94. Epub 2004/01/23.

[52] Kumar AR, Kaplowitz PB. Patient age, race and the type of diabetes have an impact on the presenting symptoms, latency before diagnosis and laboratory abnormalities at time of diagnosis of diabetes mellitus in children. Journal of clinical research in pediatric endocrinology. 2009;1(5):227-32. Epub 2009/09/01.

[53] Levy-Marchal C, Papoz L, de Beaufort C, Doutreix J, Froment V, Voirin J, et al. Clinical and laboratory features of type 1 diabetic children at the time of diagnosis. Diabetic medicine : a journal of the British Diabetic Association. 1992;9(3):279-84. Epub 1992/04/01.

[54] Pinkey JH, Bingley PJ, Sawtell PA, Dunger DB, Gale EA. Presentation and progress of childhood diabetes mellitus: a prospective population-based study. The Bart's-Oxford Study Group. Diabetologia. 1994;37(1):70-4. Epub 1994/01/01.

[55] Roche EF, Menon A, Gill D, Hoey H. Clinical presentation of type 1 diabetes. Pediatric diabetes. 2005;6(2):75-8. Epub 2005/06/21.

[56] Wolfsdorf J, Glaser N, Sperling MA, American Diabetes A. Diabetic ketoacidosis in infants, children, and adolescents: A consensus statement from the American Diabetes Association. Diabetes care. 2006;29(5):1150-9. Epub 2006/04/29.

[57] Koves IH, Neutze J, Donath S, Lee W, Werther GA, Barnett P, et al. The accuracy of clinical assessment of dehydration during diabetic ketoacidosis in childhood. Diabetes care. 2004;27(10):2485-7. Epub 2004/09/29.

[58] Edge JA, Roy Y, Bergomi A, Murphy NP, Ford-Adams ME, Ong KK, et al. Conscious level in children with diabetic ketoacidosis is related to severity of acidosis and not to blood glucose concentration. Pediatric diabetes. 2006;7(1):11-5. Epub 2006/02/24.

[59] Wolfsdorf JI, Allgrove J, Craig ME, Edge J, Glaser N, Jain V, et al. Diabetic ketoacidosis and hyperglycemic hyperosmolar state. Pediatric diabetes. 2014;15 Suppl 20:154-79. Epub 2014/07/22.

[60] Adrogue HJ, Eknoyan G, Suki WK. Diabetic ketoacidosis: role of the kidney in the acid-base homeostasis re-evaluated. Kidney international. 1984;25(4):591-8. Epub 1984/04/01.

[61] Weisberg LS. Pseudohyponatremia: a reappraisal. The American journal of medicine. 1989;86(3):315-8. Epub 1989/03/01.

[62] Kebler R, McDonald FD, Cadnapaphornchai P. Dynamic changes in serum phosphorus levels in diabetic ketoacidosis. The American journal of medicine. 1985;79(5): 571-6. Epub 1985/11/01.

[63] Carlotti AP, Bohn D, Jankiewicz N, Kamel KS, Davids MR, Halperin ML. A hyperglycaemic hyperosmolar state in a young child: diagnostic insights from a quantitative analysis. QJM : monthly journal of the Association of Physicians. 2007;100(2): 125-37. Epub 2007/02/06.

[64] Rewers A. Current concepts and controversies in prevention and treatment of diabetic ketoacidosis in children. Current diabetes reports. 2012;12(5):524-32. Epub 2012/08/07.

[65] Clark MG, Dalabih A. Variability of DKA Management Among Pediatric Emergency Room and Critical Care Providers: A Call for More Evidence-Based and Cost-Effective Care? Journal of clinical research in pediatric endocrinology. 2014;6(3):190-1. Epub 2014/09/23.

[66] Harris GD, Fiordalisi I, Yu C. Maintaining normal intracranial pressure in a rabbit model during treatment of severe diabetic ketoacidemia. Life sciences. 1996;59(20): 1695-702. Epub 1996/01/01.

[67] Clements RS, Jr., Blumenthal SA, Morrison AD, Winegrad AI. Increased cerebrospinal-fluid pressure during treatment of diabetic ketosis. Lancet. 1971;2(7726):671-5. Epub 1971/09/25.

[68] Mahoney CP, Vlcek BW, DelAguila M. Risk factors for developing brain herniation during diabetic ketoacidosis. Pediatric neurology. 1999;21(4):721-7. Epub 1999/12/02.

[69] Edge JA, Jakes RW, Roy Y, Hawkins M, Winter D, Ford-Adams ME, et al. The UK case-control study of cerebral oedema complicating diabetic ketoacidosis in children. Diabetologia. 2006;49(9):2002-9. Epub 2006/07/19.

[70] Glaser N, Barnett P, McCaslin I, Nelson D, Trainor J, Louie J, et al. Risk factors for cerebral edema in children with diabetic ketoacidosis. The Pediatric Emergency Medicine Collaborative Research Committee of the American Academy of Pediatrics. The New England journal of medicine. 2001;344(4):264-9. Epub 2001/02/15.

[71] Mel JM, Werther GA. Incidence and outcome of diabetic cerebral oedema in childhood: are there predictors? Journal of paediatrics and child health. 1995;31(1):17-20. Epub 1995/02/01.

[72] Felner EI, White PC. Improving management of diabetic ketoacidosis in children. Pediatrics. 2001;108(3):735-40. Epub 2001/09/05.

[73] Adrogue HJ, Barrero J, Eknoyan G. Salutary effects of modest fluid replacement in the treatment of adults with diabetic ketoacidosis. Use in patients without extreme volume deficit. Jama. 1989;262(15):2108-13. Epub 1989/10/20.

[74] Oh MS, Carroll HJ, Uribarri J. Mechanism of normochloremic and hyperchloremic acidosis in diabetic ketoacidosis. Nephron. 1990;54(1):1-6. Epub 1990/01/01.

[75] Fort P, Waters SM, Lifshitz F. Low-dose insulin infusion in the treatment of diabetic ketoacidosis: bolus versus no bolus. The Journal of pediatrics. 1980;96(1):36-40. Epub 1980/01/01.

[76] Lindsay R, Bolte RG. The use of an insulin bolus in low-dose insulin infusion for pediatric diabetic ketoacidosis. Pediatric emergency care. 1989;5(2):77-9. Epub 1989/06/01.

[77] Kitabchi AE. Low-dose insulin therapy in diabetic ketoacidosis: fact or fiction? Diabetes/metabolism reviews. 1989;5(4):337-63. Epub 1989/06/01.

[78] Nallasamy K, Jayashree M, Singhi S, Bansal A. Low-dose vs standard-dose insulin in pediatric diabetic ketoacidosis: a randomized clinical trial. JAMA pediatrics. 2014;168(11):999-1005. Epub 2014/09/30.

[79] Vincent M, Nobecourt E. Treatment of diabetic ketoacidosis with subcutaneous insulin lispro: a review of the current evidence from clinical studies. Diabetes & metabolism. 2013;39(4):299-305. Epub 2013/05/07.

[80] Barski L, Kezerle L, Zeller L, Zektser M, Jotkowitz A. New approaches to the use of insulin in patients with diabetic ketoacidosis. European journal of internal medicine. 2013;24(3):213-6. Epub 2013/02/12.

[81] Becker DJ, Brown DR, Steranka BH, Drash AL. Phosphate replacement during treatment of diabetic ketosis. Effects on calcium and phosphorus homeostasis. American journal of diseases of children. 1983;137(3):241-6. Epub 1983/03/01.

[82] Zipf WB, Bacon GE, Spencer ML, Kelch RP, Hopwood NJ, Hawker CD. Hypocalcemia, hypomagnesemia, and transient hypoparathyroidism during therapy with potassium phosphate in diabetic ketoacidosis. Diabetes care. 1979;2(3):265-8. Epub 1979/05/01.

[83] Morris LR, Murphy MB, Kitabchi AE. Bicarbonate therapy in severe diabetic ketoacidosis. Annals of internal medicine. 1986;105(6):836-40. Epub 1986/12/01.

[84] Green SM, Rothrock SG, Ho JD, Gallant RD, Borger R, Thomas TL, et al. Failure of adjunctive bicarbonate to improve outcome in severe pediatric diabetic ketoacidosis. Annals of emergency medicine. 1998;31(1):41-8. Epub 1998/01/23.

[85] Hale PJ, Crase J, Nattrass M. Metabolic effects of bicarbonate in the treatment of diabetic ketoacidosis. British medical journal. 1984;289(6451):1035-8. Epub 1984/10/20.

[86] Okuda Y, Adrogue HJ, Field JB, Nohara H, Yamashita K. Counterproductive effects of sodium bicarbonate in diabetic ketoacidosis. The Journal of clinical endocrinology and metabolism. 1996;81(1):314-20. Epub 1996/01/01.

[87] Assal JP, Aoki TT, Manzano FM, Kozak GP. Metabolic effects of sodium bicarbonate in management of diabetic ketoacidosis. Diabetes. 1974;23(5):405-11. Epub 1974/05/01.

[88] Ohman JL, Jr., Marliss EB, Aoki TT, Munichoodappa CS, Khanna VV, Kozak GP. The cerebrospinal fluid in diabetic ketoacidosis. The New England journal of medicine. 1971;284(6):283-90. Epub 1971/02/11.

[89] Glaser N. Cerebral edema in children with diabetic ketoacidosis. Current diabetes reports. 2001;1(1):41-6. Epub 2003/05/24.

[90] Duck SC, Kohler E. Cerebral edema in diabetic ketoacidosis. The Journal of pediatrics. 1981;98(4):674-6. Epub 1981/04/01.

[91] Glaser NS, Wootton-Gorges SL, Marcin JP, Buonocore MH, Dicarlo J, Neely EK, et al. Mechanism of cerebral edema in children with diabetic ketoacidosis. The Journal of pediatrics. 2004;145(2):164-71. Epub 2004/08/04.

[92] Glaser NS, Marcin JP, Wootton-Gorges SL, Buonocore MH, Rewers A, Strain J, et al. Correlation of clinical and biochemical findings with diabetic ketoacidosis-related cerebral edema in children using magnetic resonance diffusion-weighted imaging. The Journal of pediatrics. 2008;153(4):541-6. Epub 2008/07/01.

[93] Vavilala MS, Marro KI, Richards TL, Roberts JS, Curry P, Pihoker C, et al. Change in mean transit time, apparent diffusion coefficient, and cerebral blood volume during pediatric diabetic ketoacidosis treatment. Pediatric critical care medicine : a journal of the Society of Critical Care Medicine and the World Federation of Pediatric Intensive and Critical Care Societies. 2011;12(6):e344-9. Epub 2011/04/26.

[94] Lawrence SE, Cummings EA, Gaboury I, Daneman D. Population-based study of incidence and risk factors for cerebral edema in pediatric diabetic ketoacidosis. The Journal of pediatrics. 2005;146(5):688-92. Epub 2005/05/05.

[95] Watts W, Edge JA. How can cerebral edema during treatment of diabetic ketoacidosis be avoided? Pediatric diabetes. 2014;15(4):271-6. Epub 2014/05/29.

[96] Marcin JP, Glaser N, Barnett P, McCaslin I, Nelson D, Trainor J, et al. Factors associated with adverse outcomes in children with diabetic ketoacidosis-related cerebral edema. The Journal of pediatrics. 2002;141(6):793-7. Epub 2002/12/04.

[97] Paton RC. Haemostatic changes in diabetic coma. Diabetologia. 1981;21(3):172-7. Epub 1981/09/01.

[98]   Elding Larsson H, Vehik K, Bell R, Dabelea D, Dolan L, Pihoker C, et al. Reduced prevalence of diabetic ketoacidosis at diagnosis of type 1 diabetes in young children participating in longitudinal follow-up. Diabetes care. 2011;34(11):2347-52. Epub 2011/10/06.

[99]   Diabetes Prevention Trial--Type 1 Diabetes Study G. Effects of insulin in relatives of patients with type 1 diabetes mellitus. The New England journal of medicine. 2002;346(22):1685-91. Epub 2002/05/31.

[100] Vanelli M, Chiari G, Lacava S, Iovane B. Campaign for diabetic ketoacidosis prevention still effective 8 years later. Diabetes care. 2007;30(4):e12. Epub 2007/03/30.

[101] Vanelli M, Chiari G, Ghizzoni L, Costi G, Giacalone T, Chiarelli F. Effectiveness of a prevention program for diabetic ketoacidosis in children. An 8-year study in schools and private practices. Diabetes care. 1999;22(1):7-9. Epub 1999/05/20.

[102] King BR, Howard NJ, Verge CF, Jack MM, Govind N, Jameson K, et al. A diabetes awareness campaign prevents diabetic ketoacidosis in children at their initial presentation with type 1 diabetes. Pediatric diabetes. 2012;13(8):647-51. Epub 2012/07/24.

[103] Hoffman WH, O'Neill P, Khoury C, Bernstein SS. Service and education for the insulin-dependent child. Diabetes care. 1978;1(5):285-8. Epub 1978/09/01.

[104] Drozda DJ, Dawson VA, Long DJ, Freson LS, Sperling MA. Assessment of the effect of a comprehensive diabetes management program on hospital admission rates of children with diabetes mellitus. The Diabetes educator. 1990;16(5):389-93. Epub 1990/09/01.

[105] Grey M, Boland EA, Davidson M, Li J, Tamborlane WV. Coping skills training for youth with diabetes mellitus has long-lasting effects on metabolic control and quality of life. The Journal of pediatrics. 2000;137(1):107-13. Epub 2000/07/13.

[106] Beck JK, Logan KJ, Hamm RM, Sproat SM, Musser KM, Everhart PD, et al. Reimbursement for pediatric diabetes intensive case management: a model for chronic diseases? Pediatrics. 2004;113(1 Pt 1):e47-50. Epub 2004/01/02.

[107] Harris MA, Wagner DV, Heywood M, Hoehn D, Bahia H, Spiro K. Youth repeatedly hospitalized for DKA: proof of concept for novel interventions in children's healthcare (NICH). Diabetes care. 2014;37(6):e125-6. Epub 2014/05/24.

[108] Golden MP, Herrold AJ, Orr DP. An approach to prevention of recurrent diabetic ketoacidosis in the pediatric population. The Journal of pediatrics. 1985;107(2):195-200. Epub 1985/08/01.

[109] Laffel LM, Wentzell K, Loughlin C, Tovar A, Moltz K, Brink S. Sick day management using blood 3-hydroxybutyrate (3-OHB) compared with urine ketone monitoring reduces hospital visits in young people with T1DM: a randomized clinical trial. Diabetic medicine : a journal of the British Diabetic Association. 2006;23(3):278-84. Epub 2006/02/24.

4

Pathogenesis of
Type 2 Diabetes Mellitus

Fuad AlSaraj

1. Introduction

The natural history of type 2 diabetes (T2DM) has been well described in multiple populations. Patients with T2DM have inherited genes from parents that make their tissues resistant to insulin. Insulin resistance (IR) in muscle and liver and β-cell failure represent the core pathophysiologic defects in development of T2DM. Age, genes, IR, lipotoxicity, glucotoxicity, amyloid deposition and abnormal incretin are factors playing a role in progressive β-cells dysfunction. The progressive decline in insulin secretion, decrease of the pancreatic β- cell mass and function and the presence of IR will contribute in changing the state of the dysglycemia from normal to, impaired fasting glucose (IFG), impaired glucose tolerance (IGT) and end with overt diabetes [1].

2. Glucose metabolism

Excessive hepatic glucose output is an important factor in the fasting hyperglycemia of patients with T2DM. Following administration of isotope in healthy subjects and in patients with T2DM, the overall hepatic glucose output was an increase by twofold and the gluconeogenesis more than threefold in patients compare with the controls. This finding demonstrated the increased in gluconeogenesis is the predominant mechanism responsible for increased hepatic glucose output in patients with T2DM and it is correlated with fasting plasma glucose level. [2]. Insulin controls the hepatic glucose production and promotes glucose utilization by the skeletal muscle. There is a correlation between the hepatic glucose production and the fasting glucose, in normal subjects, the postabsorptive hepatic glucose production is increased. But in patients with T2DM, the main causes are increased mostly by gluconeogenesis and to less extent by glycogenolysis by the liver. The Increased production of gluconeogenic precursors (lactate, alanine, and glycerol) and hyperglucagonemia with increased hepatic FFA acid oxidation might be responsible for glucogenesis. There is also a reduction in suppression of hepatic glucose production after carbohydrate ingestion which plays a role in the impairment in postprandial glucose homeostasis in T2DM [3].

The increased of the glycogenolysis and the decreased in the hepatic glucose uptake by glucagon will produce hyperglycemic phenotype associated with insulin deficiency and IR. In the overnight fasted, it is essential in countering the suppressive effects of basal insulin to maintain appropriate levels of glycogenolysis, fasting hepatic glucose production and blood glucose. Glycogenolysis is also increased by the counter-regulatory hormones response to hypoglycemia and in exercise [4]. Insulin and glucagon secretion are determined by plasma glucose concentration which is widely fluctuated according to the demand such as exercise and supply as taking high carbohydrate meal. In the resting postabsorptive state, the glycogenolysis and gluconeogenesis are equal or in balance in hepatic glucose release. This is a key regulated process. In the postprandial state, suppression of liver glucose output and stimulation of skeletal muscle glucose uptake are the most important factors. Under stressful conditions, the counter-regulatory hormones of the hypoglycemia secretion are increased with increased of the sympathetic nervous system activity. Their actions to increase hepatic glucose output and to suppress tissue glucose uptake are partly mediated by increases in tissue fatty acid oxidation. In T2DM, the fasting hyperglycaemia resulted from increased gluconeogenesis while, the postprandial hyperglycemia occurs due to impaired suppression of glycogenolysis and impaired skeletal muscle glucose uptake [5].

In normal subjects the fasting plasma glucose levels are constant from day to day. This constancy is due to a close co-ordination between glucose production by the liver and glucose uptake in peripheral tissues. In T2DM, fasting hyperglycemia to less extent is correlated with increased hepatic glucose production due to impaired hepatic sensitivity to insulin. But, it is largely due to reduced insulin secretion and increased glucagon secretion. Though the basal immunoreactive insulin and glucagon levels in patients with T2DM may appear normal compared with the normal subjects, the islet function testing at matched glucose levels reveals impairments of the basal, steady-state, and stimulated insulin and glucagon secretion due to a reduction in β- cells secretory capacity and a reduced ability of glucose to suppress glucagon release. Islet α- and β-cells functions are reduced by more than 50% in T2DM by the time that clinical fasting hyperglycemia develops (140 mg/dL) [6]. The efficiency of glucose uptake by the peripheral tissues is also impaired due to a combination of decreased insulin secretion and defective of the cellular insulin action [6, 7]. The defective in first phase glucose induced insulin secretion is followed by fasting hyperglycemia and the progressive failure in pancreatic β-cells function is matched by rising glucose levels to maintain basal and second-phase insulin output. The glucose is not only directly regulated insulin synthesis and secretion. But, moderated all other islet signals, including other substrates, hormones, and neural factors. In T2DM the defects are in first-phase insulin secretion and in the deficiency of the ability of glucose to potentiate other islet nonglucose β-cell secretagogues. In T2DM patients, the resulting hyperglycemia does not correct the first phase of insulin secretion defect. However, it compensates for the defective glucose potentiation, maintains nearly normal basal insulin levels and insulin responses to nonglucose secretagogues [8].

The major primary reduction of suppression in the output of the endogenous hepatic glucose release and the minor effect of the splanchnic glucose sequestration in these patients are the cause of increasing in systemic glucose delivery which subsequently responsible for the postprandial hyperglycemia [9, 10].

The fasting hyperglycemia is mainly caused by the increased of the released hepatic glucose production. This mechanism is increased in psotabsorptive state and exhibits a positive correlation with fasting glucose level [3, 7 11].

The increase of the glucogenesis in the postprandial state represents the primary mechanism responsible for impaired suppression of hepatic glucose production [3]. The increased in the rate of glucose release by the liver results in part from impaired hepatic sensitivity to insulin, but it is largely due to reduced insulin secretion and increased glucagon secretion [6]. The degree of fasting hyperglycemia in a given patient with T2DM is closely related to the degree of impaired pancreatic β-cells responsiveness to glucose.

The fasting insulin secretion in normal subject and in patients with T2DM is comparable. But, there is a marked impairment of insulin secretion in patients with DM in relation to the degree of hyperglycemia. This is demonstrating the closed feedback loop operating between glucose levels and pancreatic β-cells which regulates the relationship of insulin secretion and hepatic glucose production [11]. The glucose uptake by peripheral tissue is impaired due to a combination of decreased insulin secretion and defective in cellular insulin action [6, 7].

The amyloid deposition process is associated with disproportionate hyperproinsulinemia. The amylin in transgenic mice develops islet amyloid deposits and hyperglycemia. This is suggestive the process of amyloid fibril formation impairs the function of the β-cells and eventual death. The progressive loss of β-cell function in T2DM, initially reflected by the loss in first-phase insulin secretion, followed by a decrease in the maximal capacity of glucose to potentiate all non-glucose signals. Finally, a defective steady-state and basal insulin secretion develops, leading to complete β-cells failure requiring insulin therapy [12].

The conclusion is, T2DM is characterized by a steady-state re-regulation of plasma glucose concentration at an elevated level in which islet cells dysfunction play a necessary role [7].

3. Insulin secretion, function and impairment

Insulin is synthesized and produced by β- cells in the pancreas. It is a peptide hormone regulates the metabolism of fat and carbohydrate in the body. It helps glucose absorption from the circulation by fat tissue and skeletal muscles. Figures 1 [13] and 2 [14].

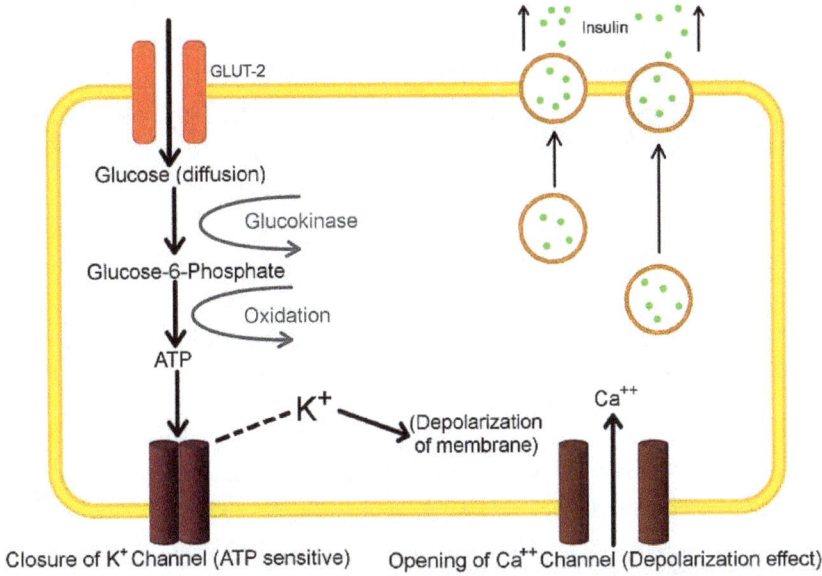

Figure 1. Insulin secretion [13].

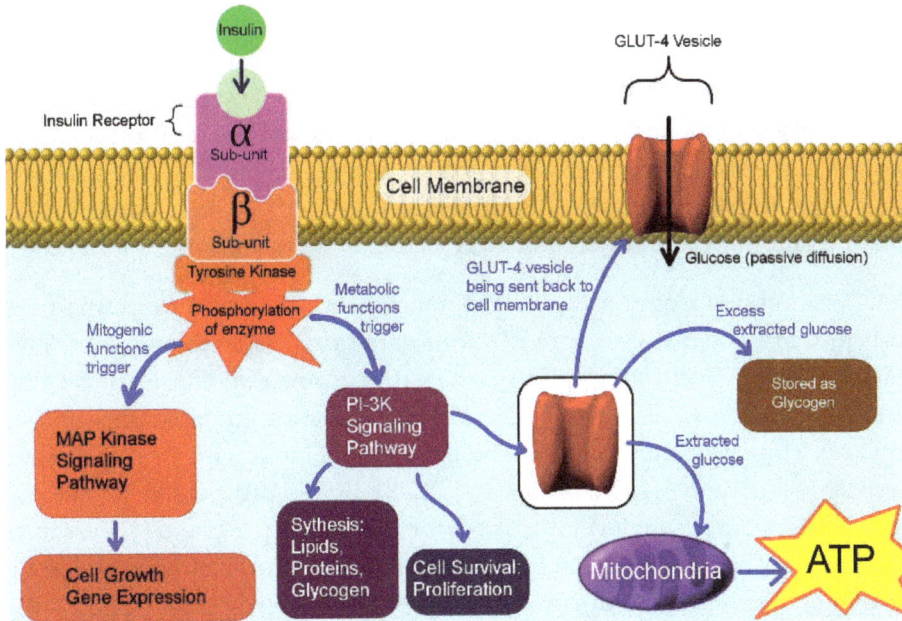

Figure 2. Insulin functions [14].

Pancreatic β-cells secrete insulin in two phases, first and second phase (biphasic manner). The loss of first phase is an independent predictor of T2DM onset. In patients with T2DM, the restoration of this phase suppresses the hepatic glucose output and improves the blood glucose concentration [15]. There are many metabolic abnormalities precede the clinical picture of

T2DM as demonstrated in a study of normal first- degree subjects who had relatives with T2DM. Following intravenous glucose infusion, these subjects showed a reduced first phase insulin secretion with decreased ability of the β-cells to respond to successive increase or decrease in glucose with mild elevation in 2hours post challenge glucose level [16]. In patients with T2DM, the earliest detectable defect and exhaustion of β- cells function appeared in the reduction of the first-phase insulin secretion. This phase is brief burst and spike lasting for about 10 minutes followed by plateau second phase lasted for 2-3 hours. The reductions in both phases occur equally early and precede development of IR [17]. The fasting plasma insulin concentration is often a marker of insulin sensitivity (IS) and the changing in acute insulin secretion following glucose challenge is an early observation of progressive pancreatic defect. Glucotoxicity and lipototoxicity are contributor factors in progressive and the continuous decline in pancreatic function [1, 18].

Insulin is secreted from the secretory cells by priming reaction. Each cell contains thousands of secretory vesicles/granules. Less than <5% of these cells exist to release the readily pool insulin by exocytosis followed by minimal latency of immediate releasable pool of insulin. The bulk of granules in the cell (>95%) exist in a non-releasable reserve pool of insulin, which must undergo a series of ATP-, Ca^{2+}-, and temperature-dependent reactions to release insulin [19].

The prevalence of Gestational diabetes (GDM) is 2-3% of all pregnant women. GDM women have the same second –phase insulin response as women with normal oral GTT. But, the first phase-insulin secretion is reduced with intravenous glucose and has a later peak rise with OGTT. Both groups showed a decreased in IS by 50-70%, this is back to normal in postpartum period in women with normal OGTT but this is not in women with GDM. In the same period, the latter group also demonstrated a persistent and excessive proinsulin secretion. Women with GDM have also a substantial increase in insulin secretion with OGTT or a meal compared to the same women in postpartum period. But this rise is less in women with GDM compared with pregnant women who retain normal OGTT [20].

The glycemic progression from normal to IGT mainly due to IR and from this state to overt DM depends primarily on β-cells failure in addition to progression to severe IR. Two studies, San Antonio and Hoorn Study showed the high fasting proinsulin reflects the β-cells dysfunction and the progression to DM. IR is determined by fasting hyperinsulinemia and lower glucose removal. Therefore, the 2 hours blood glucose level following oral glucose load is the most powerful in prediction of development of T2DM. IR and progressive β-cells dysfunction are the two important defects in development of the disease [21]. IFG and IGT are intermediate states in glucose metabolism that exist between normal GT and overt diabetes are related to these defects in addition to the reduction in early-phase insulin secretion. But, subjects with IGT also have impaired late-phase insulin secretion. The latter group also demonstrated a significant higher muscle IR and low hepatic IR while subjects with IFG have severe hepatic IR with normal or near-normal muscle IS [22]. The insulin secretion and glucose homeostasis in the first phaase insulin secretion is determined by a complex pathawy of multiple signals including hypoxia inducible factor 1α, von Hippel-Lindau, factor inhibiting HIF, nicotinamide phospho-ribosyl-transferase, and the sirtuin family in addition to many other novel regulatory factors are crucial [15].

4. Insulin resistance

Patients with T2DM have high whole body glucose production and glucogenesis but low glycogenolysis compared with normal subjects. In patients with IR, there is impairment of glucose transport and insulin signaling in target tissues with release of inflammatory markers from the adipose tissue [23, 24]. The glucose, FFA, autonomic nerves, fat-derived hormones and the gut hormone glucagon-like peptide-1 (GLP-1) are mediators sending signals to the β-cells to respond to IR. The maintenance of normal glucose and lipid metabolism is by the reciprocal relation of IR to IS and insulin secretion. Hyperbolic relation is the best description of the curvilinear relation between IS and secretion. This relation is impaired with failure of these signals to act on β-cells to secret insulin ends with subsequent development of dysglycemia (Impaired Fasting glucose- IFG, impaired Glucose tolerance –IGT and DM) [25].

Obesity is the most common cause of IR and T2DM. Simply being overweight (BMI >25) raises the risk of developing T2DM by a factor of 3 [26].

The main components of IR are dysglycemia, dyslipidemia, obesity, hypertension and hyperinsulinemia. Therefore, it is the key feature of metabolic syndrome (MS) and vascular complications (cardiovascular and stroke). IR components once are acquired, those with genetic predisposition will develop the full picture of the disorder suggesting the final phenotypic expression involves both genetic and acquired influences. The most important environmental factor in IR is central obesity which is mainly caused by intake of high fat, and refined carbohydrate without physical activity. These are exacerbated by genetic predisposition but IR could be reduced with minimizing dietary intake and regular exercise [27].

The three potential mechanisms of the controlling glucose metabolism in the skeletal muscles are the glycogen synthase, the hexokinase and the major insulin-stimulated glucose transporter GLUT4. Therefore, defects in glycogen synthesis in the skeletal muscles playing a major role in the pathogenesis of IR [28]. The decrease in the ability of normal responding skeletal muscles to circulating insulin levels or concentrations is main principle of development of IR which could precede the overt T2DM by 10 to 20years [28].

T2DM is characterized by increased hepatic glucose output, increased peripheral resistance to insulin action (due to receptor and postreceptor defects) and impaired insulin secretion.

Two major variants of insulin receptor abnormalities associated with acanthosis nigricans, hyperinsulinemia and marked hyperandrogenism. The classic type A IR syndrome, which is due to genetic defect in the insulin-signaling system such as mutation in the insulin receptor gene [29] and type B IR syndrome, which results from autoantibodies to the insulin receptor [30].

Many factors could enhance IR include, obesity, inflammation and inflammatory markers, defects in genes and drugs. These will be demonstrated further in this chapter.

5. The role of obesity and inflammatory markers in insulin resistance and T2DM

Obesity has a substantial negative effect on life expectancy and longevity. It reduces the length of life in severely obese people by an estimation of 5 to 20 years. This negative effect should be addressed in the health public policy [31]. Obesity, IR, and T2DM are growing health concerns, and the incidence and the prevalence of these diseases are increasing worldwide [32, 33]. Obesity will cause a decline in life expectancy for the first time in recent history due to numerous co-morbid disorders [31] and it is a risk factor for many human diseases [34]. Obesity is associated with an increased risk of developing IR and T2DM [34, 35]. The primary defects in obese individuals are the dysfunction of adipocyte and adipose tissue [34].

IR in obese subjects is determined by the release of high amounts of non-esterified FA, glycerol, hormones, pro-inflammatory cytokines and many other factors from adipose or fat tissue. This is followed by dysfunction of pancreatic β- cells and failure to secret insulin to control blood glucose levels. These metabolic and inflammatory changes are critical in defining the risk and the development of T2DM. [35]. There is a clear hyperbolic relationship between IS and insulin secretion by the β-cells of the pancreas. This demonstrates the concept of a feedback loop governs the interaction between the β-cells function and IS tissues. This helpful in explain that patients or subjects with IR have significant increase in insulin response compared with low responses in IS group [11, 36].

IR is a characteristic feature of T2DM and obesity, and the majority of patients with T2DM are obese. Obesity has a major impact to cause IR in subjects without DM. IR is the primary defect in obese elderly and middle aged patients with T2DM despite, adequate circulating insulin. But, in the second group the impairment of insulin release and the alteration of hepatic glucose output are other defects contributing to the development of the disease [37, 38, 39]. The intra-abdominal fat is a major determinant of IR among other distributed fat in the body while the dysfunction of the β- cells is correlated with reduction of β-cells mass and subsequently reduction in IS. The genetic and the molecular basis of these pathological abnormalities are there. But, not fully understood. As mentioned, the progressive declining or failure of the β-cells function and IS are associated with development of T2DM. Prior to the onset of T2DM, there are stages from normal glucose concentration to dysglycemia (IFG, IGT) emphasizing in number of ethnic group the OGTT response is a major determinant of β-cells function [25, 36]. The elevations in plasma FFA concentrations in obese subjects and in patients with T2DM inhibit insulin stimulated peripheral glucose uptake (fat and skeletal muscle) and glycogen synthesis [40, 41].

The impairment of adipose tissue functions in obese subjects caused by interaction of genetic and environmental factors and subsequently leads to obesity medical co-morbidities. However, not all obese patients develop the same complications. The adipocyte dysfunctions or impairment occur in form of ectopic fat deposition, adipocyte hypertrophy, hypoxia, changes in the cellular composition with a variety of stresses and inflammatory processes in the fat tissue (release a proinflammatory, atherogenic, and diabetogenic adipokine pattern), increased lipid storage and impaired IS [33]. Obese individuals have large or expanded fat mass and have high or elevated plasma concentration fatty acids [42, 43, 44].

Glucose uptake rather than intracellular glucose metabolism has been implicated as the rate-limiting step for FA-induced IR [45].

In adipose tissue, the glucocorticoids can be produced locally from inactive 11-keto forms through the enzyme 11beta hydroxysteroid dehydrogenase type 1 (11beta HSD-1). In obese human, the glucocorticoids are normal. However, the excess of glucocorticoids produce visceral obesity, IR and DM. In mice, the transgenic mice overexpressing 11beta HSD-1 selectively in adipose tissue was exaggerated by high fat diet showed an increase in the level of corticosterone in adipose tissue by increased adipocyte 11beta HSD-1 activity. This could have the same effect in human[46] suggesting that increases in endogenous 11β-HSD1 in the adipose tissue of obese humans and rodents [47,48] contribute to obesity-associated IR, in part due to increased delivery of glucocorticoids to the liver via the portal vein. The c-Jun amino-terminal kinases (JNKs) interfere with insulin action and it is crucial mediator of obesity and IR. In obese mouse, the JNK activity is abnormally elevated and the absence of JNK1 results in decreased adiposity and improved IS. Therefore, it is a potential target for therapeutics [49].

The activation of JNK1 leads to serine phosphorylation of IRS-1 that impairs insulin action [50, 51]. In addition, IKK-β is a mediator of TNF-induced IR [52, 53, 54, 55] demonstrated the TLR4 (Lipopolysaccharide receptor) activation by FFA, plays a critical role in innate immunity and IR in obese human and animals through activation of inflammatory pathways. In mice the lack of TLR4 will protect insulin suppression signaling and reduce insulin mediated changes in systemic glucose metabolism by lipid infusion. This indicates the effect of nutrition as environmental factor on TLR4 and subsequently on IR. The Apoptosis signal-regulating kinase 1 (ASK1) is an evolutionarily conserved mitogen-activated protein 3-kinase that activates both Jnk and p38 mitogen-activated protein kinases. The reactive oxygen species-dependent TRAF6-ASK1-p38 axis is crucial for TLR4-mediated mammalian innate immunity [53, 54]. This finding may provide an additional link between innate immunity, cellular stress, and IR. The protein tyrosine phosphatase receptor T (PTPRT) knockout mice are resistant to high-fat diet-induced obesity. The PTPRT-modulated STAT3 signaling in the regulation of high-fat diet-induced obesity [34]. Figures 3 and 4 with Table 1.

Adipokine	Distribution	Function	Effect in obesity
Leptin	Secreted predominantly by WAT, to lesser degree, in ypothalamus, gastric epithelium, placenta & gonads.	Regulates energy intake, expenditure & feeding behavior. Also regulates storage of fat & insulin signaling.	↑ in mouse models of obesity. ↑ in human obesity & correlated with BMI & ↓ in weight loss.
Adiponektin	Secreted exclusively by adipocytes. mRNA & protein in Sc AT > Omental AT.	Improves energy homeostasis, IS & Glucose uptake. Anti-Inflammatory properties.	↓ in mouse models of obesity and IR (ob/ob and db/db).

Adipokine	Distribution	Function	Effect in obesity
	2–3 times greater secretion in females.		↓ in human obesity & T2DM patients. ↑ after weight loss
Resistin	In rodents, secreted by adipocytes. In humans, secreted predominantly by circulating macrophages & monocytes, to a lesser degree, by WAT.	Implicated in glucose metabolism, in the regulation of gluconeogenesis & IR in rodents. More roinflammatory role in humans.	↑ circulating concentrations in mouse models of obesity. ↑ in human obesity & correlated with IR in T2DM patients.
TNF-α	Expressed by macrophages & adipocytes (visceral WAT > subcutaneous WAT).	Affects insulin & glucose metabolism. Provokes IR & stimulates lipolysis.	↑ in mouse models of obesity. ↑ in human obesity & correlated with BMI
IL-6	One-third of total circulating levels are expressed predominantly by adipocytes. Also expressed in macrophages, skeletal muscle, endothelial cells & fibroblasts.	Controversial role in the development of IR. Affects glucose metabolism	↑ circulating levels in human obese subjects & correlated with adiposity & reduced with weight loss. ↑ in plasma of T2DM patients.
IL-7	Secreted by stromal & vascular endothelial cells.	Homeostatic immune cytokine. Also regulates body weight, AT mass & function, and insulin signaling.	↑ in morbidly obese subjects.
IL-8	Secreted by adipocytes (visceral WAT > SC WAT) & macrophages.	Neutrophil chemotaxis.	↑ in obese subjects & related to fat mass & TNF-α levels.
IL-1	Secreted mainly by adipocytes & macrophages.	Role in macrophages chemotaxis & thermogenesis	↑ in obese mice. ↑ in human obesity & predictive of T2DM.
IL-10	Secreted by monocytes, macrophages, dendritic cells, B & T cells.	Improves IS & glucose transport.	Attenuated in T2DM patients & ↑ with weight loss
RBP4	Secreted by adipocytes, macrophages & hepatocytes.	Affects IS, hepatic glucose output & muscle insulin signaling.	↑ circulating levels in obese subjects & correlated with BMI & IR.
MCP-1	Secreted by AT.	Affects IS & ↑ macrophage recruitment in AT and inflammation.	↑ in mouse models of obesity. ↑ in T2DM subjects.
PAI-1	Expressed by WAT.	Potent inhibitor of fibrinolytic pathway.	↑ in human obesity and T2DM subjects.

Adipokine	Distribution	Function	Effect in obesity
CXCL5	Secreted by macrophages within the stromal vascular fraction.	Interferes with insulin signaling in muscle.	Circulating levels are higher in obese IR individuals than in obese IS & ↓ after a 4-weeks period on low-calorie diet.
Visfatin	Expressed in liver, muscle, WAT, bone marrow & lymphocytes	Role in IS, insulin secretion & inflammatory properties.	↑ in obesity & correlates with visceral adiposity in humans.
Chemerin	In rodents & humans, expressed in placenta & WAT.	Regulates adipocyte development & metabolic function.	↑ circulating levels in obese & T2DM patients and correlated with body fat, glucose & lipid metabolism.
Vaspin	Secreted by WAT, hypothalamus, pancreatic islets & skin.	Improves IS.	↑ in obesity & T2DM patients
Omentin	Secreted by omental AT.	↑ IS	↓ in obesity.
Apelin	Produced in a wide range of tissues.	Improves IS mainly acting in skeletal muscle & adipocytes in mice.	↑ in obesity, IGT & T2DM patients. ↓ after weight loss following diet & bariatric surgery.
Nesfatin	Secreted in brain tissue, B cells and AT.	Central action to ↓ Appetite.	↓ in obesity.
TGFβ	Multifunctional, produced By variety of cells. Inhibitor of differentiation.	Varied role in proliferation, differentiation, apoptosis and development.	↑ ob/ob and db/db mice. ↑ preadipocyte cell proliferation as with TNFα. ↑ in obesity, T2DM patients & CVD.
Rantes	Pro -inflammatory secreted by T cells, monocytes & to lesser degree in WAT.	↑ gene expression in AT.	No correlation of serum level with obesity.
Preptin	It is a novel hormone that is co-secreted with insulin and amylin from pancreatic β-cells [60].	Synthetic prepin ↑ insulin secretion from glucose stimulated β TC6-F7 in a concentration- dependent and saturable manner [61].	Plasma preptin level ↑ with higher BMI [62]. It is ↑ in patients with T2DM compared with patients with IGT and normal subjects [61].
Uncoupling protein 2	It is expressed in AT, skeletal muscle and tissue of immune system [63].	It protects cell function from damage and it impairs insulin secretion from β-cells [64].	Anti-oxidant in pancreatic β-cells [65]. The level and activity has impact on glucose stimulated insulin secretion [66].

Table 1. Adipokines increased in obesity and/or diabetes [58, 59].

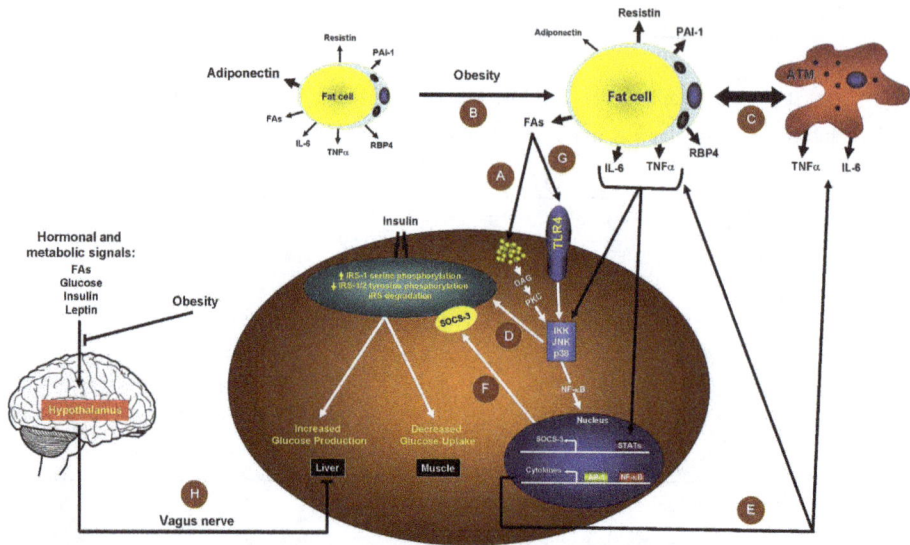

Figure 3. The molecular linked pathway between obesity and IR. (*A*) IR triggered by the increase in FAs through intra-cellular metabolites that activate PKC, leading to inhibit insulin signaling by activation of serine/threonine kinases. (*B*) Insulin signaling modulated by changes in adipokines secretion. (*C*) In the adipose tissue; the increased in the ATMs mediated the increase of the inflammatory cytokines that inhibit insulin signaling. (*D*) Insulin signaling inhibited by mediators (Endocrine and Inflammatory) converging on serine/threonine kinases. (*E*) IR exacerbated by activation of NF-κB heightens inflammatory responses. (*F*) Adipokines induced SOCS family proteins interfering with IRS-1 and IRS-2 tyrosine phosphorylation or by targeting IRS-1 and IRS-2 for proteosomal degradation inducing IR. (*G*) IR triggered by activation TLR4 and innate immune response by FAs. (*H*) Alteration in peripheral IS is related to the central response to hormonal and nutrient signals [57].

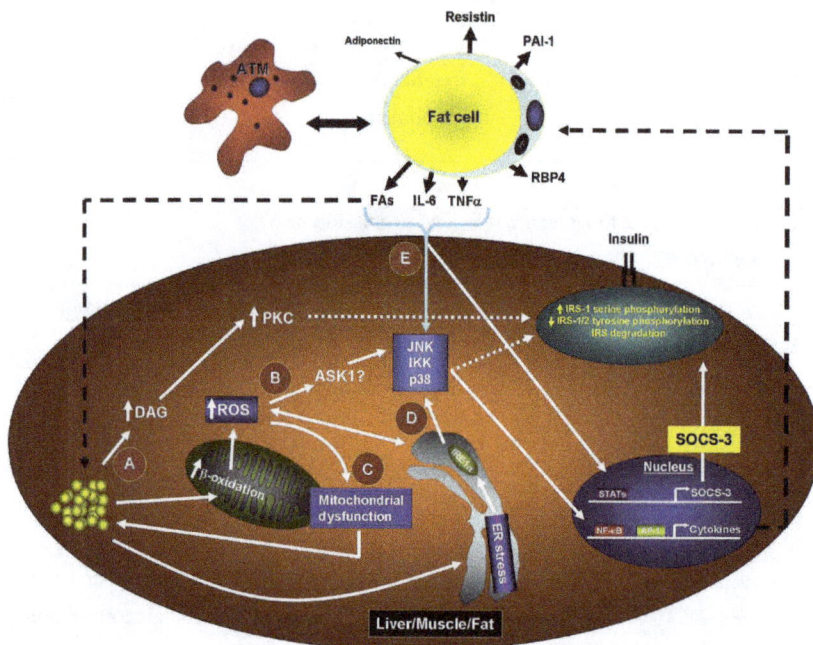

Figure 4. There are several cell-intrinsic mediators and pathways dysregulation in obesity with negative impact on IR. (*A*) Activation of PKC in the liver and muscles inhibits insulin signaling by increasing FA from ectopic adipose tissue. (*B*) Direct inhibition of insulin signaling through IRS-1 or IRS-2 serine phosphorylation or indirectly through a series of

transcriptional events mediated by NF-κB. Inhibition occurs due to activation of several serine/threoning kinases (JNK, IKK, and p38 MAPK) by excess in ROS. The later generation increased by mitochondrial β- oxidation triggered by excess fat accumulation. (C) IR exacerbated by mitochondrial dysfunction through increasing intracellular lipid accumulation. (D) Insulin signaling suppressed by activation of JNK or through a potential increase in ROS production and both activated by cellular ER stresses responses. (E) The cell-extrinsic modulators such as endocrine and inflammatory signals can intensified IR [57].

WAT: White adipose tissue, AT: adipose tissue, T2DM: type 2 diabetes mellitus, IR: insulin resistance, IS: insulin sensitivity, IGT: impaired glucose tolerance, TNF-α: tumor necrosis alpha, IL: interleukin, RBP4: Retinol binding protein, SC: subcutaneous, MCP-1: monocyte chemotactic protein 1, PAI: plasminogen activator inhibitor, CXCL5: chemokines molecules (CXCL5 ligand 5), TGFβ: transforming growth factor β.

6. Others

6.1. Glucose transporters

Glucose transporters (GLUT) are integral membrane proteins that mediate the transport of glucose and structurally-related substances across the cellular membranes [67].

Sugar transport catalyzed by 11 out of 14 members of the human GLUT family. There are specific characteristics of each isotypes. They are different in expression profile, substrate specificity and kinetic characteristics. Therefore, the tissue adaptation of the glucose uptake will be determined and regulated by specific tissue gene expression. GLUT4 malfunction in expression or regulation contributes to IR while GLU2 plays a role in hormonal and neuronal control by acting a glucose sensor in β-cells of the pancreas and neuronal cells [68]. GLUT1 is ubiquitously expressed with particularly high levels in human erythrocytes and in the endothelial cells lining the blood vessels of the brain. GLUT3 is expressed primarily in neurons and, together, GLUT1 and GLUT3 allow glucose to cross the blood-brain barrier and enter neurons [69].

The GLUTI, GLUT2, and GLUU3 are the major glucose transporters isoforms present in these cells and they are constitutively localized to the plasma membrane. The glucose flux across the membrane is largely dependent upon the circulating blood glucose level or concentration. In acute state, the glucose regulated the transport system in the muscles and fat cells responded within minutes to insulin [70].

GLUT4 is the primary hormonally-responsive transporter and it is the major insulin-responsive transporter [69]. GLUT4 expression is also reduced by low insulin states, such as in muscle during fasting, and in IR adipose tissue [71]. The malfunction of glucose transporter expression or regulation (GLUT4) appears to contribute to the IR syndrome [68].

7. Genes in type 2 Diabetes Mellitus

T2DM is a complex diseases arise from interactions of multiple genes with environmental factors. These genes are variables in strength, site of interaction and are different in general population according to race and ethnicity. The diabetes genes are involved in insulin signaling, insulin secretion, IR, glucose metabolism and obesity. In addition, T2DM could be a component of many syndromes of identified inherited genes [72]. The genetic risk for T2DM changes as humans first began migrating around the world, implying a strong environmental component has affected the genetic-basis of the disease [73, 74]. Immigrants to Western developed countries, for instance, may be more prone to diabetes as compared to its lower incidence in their countries of origins [75]. In meta-analysis of different ethnicities was included in a cross –sectional data from 16 cohorts from the DECODA (Diabetes Epidemiology: Collaborative Analysis of Diagnostic Criteria in Asia) demonstrated; the waist-to-stature ratio in Asian was stronger than BMI is associated with DM in adjusted age group in both genders [76]. In Japanese-American the prevalence of DM was reduced among the men who had retained a more Japanese lifestyle through higher levels of physical activity and consumed more carbohydrates with less fat and animal protein in their diet. An inverse association between DM and being born in Japan was observed independent of age, body mass index, physical activity, and percentages of calories from fat or carbohydrates [77]. In Fiji population the disease pattern is determined by the modern lifestyle as in many industrial counties. The increase in mortality in this population was contributing to 6% and 30% due to DM and CVD respectively [78]. In USA, the large burden of T2DM in relative to non-Latino Whites, Latinos —those of Mexican origin in particular is related to mixed acculturation to US lifestyles and with greater time living in the States [79]. This was supported by other two studies. The first showed IR, hyperinsulineamia and T2DM with secondary lipid disturbances are the possible mechanism of higher morbidity and mortality from CHD in UK immigrants from the Indian subcontinent (South Asian) than other general population independently of the dietary fat intakes, smoking, blood pressure, or plasma lipids [80]. The second study also observed IR is the common pathogenic mechanism and is a risk factor of increasing the prevalence of CHD, T2DM, low HDL and hypertriglyceridemia in first generation immigrant Asian Indian to the USA compared with native Caucasian population [81]. The two major environmental risk factors for T2DM are obesity (≥ 120% ideal body weight or a body mass index > 30 k/m^2) and the sedentary lifestyle [82, 83]. Thus, the tremendous increase in the rates of T2DM in recent years has been attributed, primarily, to the dramatic rise in obesity worldwide [84]. Obesity is a progressive disease and up to 80% of patients with T2DM and PCOS patients can be attributed to obesity. It is a progressive condition leads to medical co-morbidities which are more prevalent with age and higher BMI, particularly in those with a central obesity [85]. In Pima Indians adolescents, the prevalence of T2DM was 50.9 per 1000 in 1967-1976 increased to 6 folds in 1987-1996. In American Indian and first nation youth, T2DM was more prevalent in 10-19 years old young group. Mainly in obese subjects with acanthosis nigiricans and had family history of the disease [86]. Sinha R, reported 25% of obese children (4 to 10 years of age) and 21%t of obese adolescents (11 to 18 years of age) had IGT and 4% of the obese adolescent has silent T2DM [87]. The increase in physical activity plays an important role in reducing risk of obesity and T2DM. The prolonged TV watching is associated with a significantly increased risk of obesity and T2DM, independent of diet and exercise. Men watching TV more than 40 hours per week have threefold of increase risk of developing T2DM compared with those less than I hour TV watching. Therefore, the public health campaign of decrease sedentary life should accompany the increase in physical activity [88].

Physical activity has also been inversely related to body mass index and IGT. Interventional studies in China, Finland and the US demonstrated the decrease in the risk of incidence and in the progression from pre-diabetes stage (IGT) to T2DM by intensive lifestyle interventions targeting diet and exercise. The Finnish Diabetes Prevention Study showed a reduction by 58% and in the china study was 31% with diet and 42% with diet and exercise. This was supported by USA study showed the same risk reduction with intensive lifestyle as in the Finnish study and also a reduction of 31% with metformin indicating that lifestyle intervention is better than drugs in T2DM prevention [89, 90, 91].

Xue Sun [92] reviewed a large-scale of association studies, and the genome-wide association studies (GWAS). Both have successfully identified multiple genes that contribute to T2DM susceptibility. Linkage analysis, candidate gene approach, large-scale association studies, and GWAS have identified approximately 70 loci conferring susceptibility to T2DM. Among them, 45 loci were identified in European populations, and the other 29 loci were identified in Asian populations, especially in East and South Asians. The immediate benefit derived from these findings was the better understanding of the pathophysiology of T2DM. A great number of studies have suggested that genetic variants in or near KCNJ11, TCF7L2, WFS1, HNF1B, IGF2BP2, CDKN2ACDKN2B, CDKAL1, SLC30A8, HHEX/IDE, KCNQ1, THADA, TSPAN8/ LGR5, DC123/CAMK1D, JAZF1, MTNR1B, DGKB/TMEM195, GCK, PROX1, ADCY5, SRR, CENTD2, ST6GAL1, HNF4A, KCNK16, FITM2-R3HDML-HNF4A, GLIS3, GRB14, ANK1, BCAR1, RASGRP1, and TMEM163 may confer T2DM risk through impaired -β-cell function [93-97] whereas PPARγ, ADAMTS9, IRS1, GCKR, RBMS1/ITGB6, PTPRD, DUSP9, HMGA2, KLF14, GRB14, ANKRD55, and GRK5 have an impact on insulin action [94,98-100]. FTO and MC4R, previously identified genes associated with obesity, appear to confer T2DM risk through their primary effects on BMI, but recent GWAS have shown that their effects on T2DM were independent of BMI, though FTO may have a small but detectable influence on T2DM risk through insulin action [101,102].

Barnet AH; concluded the higher concordance rate in identical twins than in non-identical twins regardless the age of the onset of the disease and in identical twins, the concordant for DM is usually in older age group compared with the younger [103]. In Japan, The Concordance between monozygotic twins was 83% for T2DM and was 40% between dizygotic twins for T2DM. This concordance was significantly greater in monozygotic than in dizygotic twins and among twins with later onset of DM (after the age of 20) than early onset. It was also observed, the loss of the early-phase insulin response for OGTT in T2DM co-twins [104]. The role of obesity or BMI in twins as a risk of DM varies in heterogeneous genetic background. The index twins of concordant pairs had been less obese than discordant pairs. This is suggestive obesity has a role in pathogenesis of DM in those with weaker genetic susceptibility for the disease [5].

Nonetheless, non diabetes first-degree relatives of T2DM patients have an almost three fold increased lifetime risk of T2DM in comparison to the background population [106]. In other study 40% of first-degree relatives of T2DM patients develop diabetes as compared to 6% in the general population [106]. IR is an early metabolic feature of nondiabetic first-degree relatives of T2DM patients [107,108] and also shows familial clustering in keeping with an underlying genetic predisposition [109,110]. The defects of insulin action are retained in cultured skeletal muscle cells from IR subjects and T2DM patients [111,112] suggesting that genetic variation contributes to decreased insulin action. While IR is a common feature of T2DM, the severity and clinical importance varies considerably across the T2DM population [113].

7.1. Inherited DM: Maturity onset diabetes of the young or MODY

The transcription factor genes play a crucial role in the normal development and function of the β-cell. MODY is a distinct type of heterogeneous group of disorders caused by mutations in β-cell transcription factors. MODY is an autosomal dominant mode of inheritance β- cell dysfunction in young age group (usually before 25 years). It is difficult to distinguish between MODY and other forms of DM because of primary defect is pancreatic β-cell dysfunction in patients with MODY. There are at least nine mutations of different gens that result in MODY phenotypes which account in about 1-2% or 2-5% of patients diagnosed with DM (approximately 20000 in UK). The transcription factors hepatocyte nuclear factor HNF - α1, HNF-4α, insulin promoter factor (IPF)-1, HNF-1β, and NeuroD1 are the main identified genes in MODY. The Glucokinase (GCK) is an enzyme responsible for glucose phosphorylation, whereas HNF-1α, HNF-4α, IPF1, HNF-1β, and NEUROD1 are all transcription factors that modulate the expression of several genes involved in differentiation and function of β-cells. This enzyme is a key in blood glucose homeostasis and the defective in kinase gene metabolism implicated in the pathogenesis of DM. There is a linkage between the GCK locus on chromosome 7p and diabetes in 16 French families with MODY and the same linkage was demonstrated in a large 5-generation pedigree (BX) with 15 members with DM. Mutations in the GCK gene cause a mild, asymptomatic and non-progressive fasting hyperglycaemia from birth usually requiring no treatment. The gene on chromosome 7 (MODY2) encodes the glycolytic enzyme glucokinases plays a key role in generating the metabolic signal for insulin secretion and in integrating hepatic glucose uptake. Other linkage studies have localized other genes mutation in MODY on human chromosomes 20 (MODY1) and 12 (MODY3), with MODY2 and MODY3 being allelic with the genes encoding glucokinase. MODY1 is an encoding (hepatocyte nuclear factor) HNF-4α (gene symbol, TCF14), a member of the steroid/thyroid hormone receptor superfamily and an upstream regulator of HNF-1 α expression. This is a transcription factor involved in tissue-specific regulation of liver genes but also expressed in pancreatic islets, insulinoma cells and other tissues. Mutations in the GCK and HNF1- α/4-α genes account for up to 80% of all MODY cases, these mutations appear in different transcription factor genes result in different clinical presentations. Mutations in the genes encoding the transcription factors HNF-1α and HNF-4α cause a progressive insulin secretory defect and hyperglycemia while mutations in the GCK gene cause a mild and non-progressive disease. MODY3 form has also mutations in the gene encoding hepatocyte nuclear factor-1 α (HNF-1α, which is encoded by the gene TCF1). Mutations in HNF-1α are highly penetrant with 63%of mutation carriers having diabetes by the age of 25 years, 78.6% by 35 years, and 95.5% by 55 years resulted in progressive β- cell dysfunction with increasing treatment requirements, greater risk of complications with age and appear to be renal dysfunction, which is often diagnosed before diabetes. Mutations in HNF-4α result in same mode of β- cell deterioration in β-cells function but the diagnosis in the later age. Mutations in IPF-1 (PDX-1) are not a common cause of MODY. MODY1 form has mutations in the gene encoding hepatonuclear factor HNF-4 α (gene symbol, TCF14) is a member of the steroid/thyroid hormone receptor superfamily and an upstream regulator of HNF-1α expression. The deficient binding of NEUROD1 or binding of a transcriptionally inactive NEUROD1 polypeptide to target promoters in pancreatic islets leads to the development of T2DM in humans. In mice, two mutations in NEUROD1 in the heterozygous state were described in development of T2DM. The truncated polypeptide lacking the carboxy-terminal trans-activation domain, a region that associates with the co-activators CBP and p300 is more severe clinically than mutation at Arg 111 in the DNA-binding domain, abolishes E-box binding activity of NEUROD1 [114-125]. Other rare forms of MODY are CEL-MODY, ABCC8, KCNJ11 and UPD6 [126]. There are many factors determined the clinical presentation of various subtype of MODY including, the severity, the course of insulin secretion defect, the risk of microvascular complications and the presence of other abnormalities or defects in diabetes patients [127].

7.2. Mitochondrial diabetes: A monogenic Diabetes Mellitus

Maternally inherited diabetes and deafness (MIDD) is a new sub-type of diabetes with mutation in mitochondrial DNA. The mitochondrial genome is passed and inherited exclusively by maternal line. In patients with T2DM there could be increase in transmission of inherited diseases by maternal line more than paternal. However, only 0.5-2.8% of patients with DM demonstrated the frequency of adenine to guanine mutation. The adenine to guanine transition mutation at position 3243 in the dihydrouridine loop of mitochondrial tRNA$^{Leu(UUR)}$ gene is specific to patients with a neurological syndrome MELAS (myopathy, encephalopathy, lactic acidosis and stroke like disease). There is also 3243 mutation is associated with the phenotypical distinct of MIDD sub-type. In a study of the genotype of patients with T2DM of North European extraction with one or more features of MIDD and/or MELAS, Two patients were identified with the mutation giving a prevalence rate of 0.13% for the whole study population, and 0.45% for the sample with phenotypic features of MIDD. Other mitochondrial gene defects and mutation of 3234 are linked to the development of T2DM [128-133].

8. The monogenic forms of Insulin Resistance (IR)

A clear genotype-phenotype association is emerging following description of more than 60 mutations in insulin receptor gene which subsequently causing IR and tend to genera extreme and severe forms of IR patients. The most abundant mutations are heterozygous leading to decreased tyrosine phosphorylation of the β-subunit of the insulin receptor.

- Type A insulin resistance syndrome, it is a heterozygous mutations in the tyrosine kinase domain of the insulin receptor gene and it is the most common phenotype. It is characterized by acanthosis nigricans and hyperandrogenism without obesity or lipoatrophy.

- Homozygous or compound heterozygous mutations lead to the Rabson–Mendelhall syndrome with severe impairment of insulin receptor function.

- Donohue syndrome (Leprechaunism) is the most extreme form of IR in humans in whom mutations resulting in complete or near-complete absence of functional insulin receptors. [134,135,136]

- Dunnigan-type familial partial lipodystrophy (FPLD) is a rare autosomal dominant form of monogenic IR. FPLD patients are born with normal fat distribution but after the onset of puberty, they lose fat from their extremities and gluteal region. The mutation of LMNA, which encodes nuclear lamin A and C on chromosome 1q21, underlies FPLD. These patients have low leptin levels and FPDL is linked to early coronary heart disease. The LMNA codon 482 missense mutation was observed to strongly associated with hyperinsulinemia, dyslipidemia, hypertension, and T2DM [137,138,139].

- The PPARγ gene, encoding the receptor through which the insulin-sensitizing drugs, the thiazolidinediones, mediate their effects the peroxisome proliferator-activated receptor gamma (PPARγ) has become a prime candidate in the search for mutations causing IR [140]. The new missense mutations in the ligand-binding domain of PPARγ were found in family (mother and her son) was heterozygous for a single nucleotide substitution with mutation at codon P467L. The mother had history of irregular period, infertility disorder, Gestational DM followed by frank DM requiring high doses of insulin (severe IR). Her son had history of early onset T2DM and hypertension. The third subject was a young female from another family presented with primary amenorrhoea, hirsutism, acanthosis nigricans and hypertension. She was heterozygous from different mutation at codon V290 of a single nucleotide substitution. These new subtypes of dominantly inherited T2DM due to defective transcription factor function resulting in impaired insulin action rather than secretion [141]. Studies to determine if mutations in the PPARγ gene predispose to diabetes in the general population show a complex relationship.

8.1. Insulin gene

Several phenotypes, including T2DM, polycystic ovary syndrome, and birth weight are associated with tandem repeat (VNTR) minisatellite 5' of the insulin gene (INS). A study analyzed this insulin gene class III VNTR minisatellite in 155 European T2DM parent-offspring trios from the British Diabetes Association demonstrated that variation within the TH-INS-IGF2 locus, most plausibly at the VNTR itself at this regulatory element is a significant determinant of T2DM susceptibility. This susceptibility is exclusively mediated by paternally derived alleles [142].

8.1.1. SUR-1gene

In Dutch population, the exon 16-3t allele of the single nucleotide polymorphisms in the sulphonylurea receptor gene (SUR1) has been reported to be associated with T2DM patients compared with the control group. But there was no association between T2DM patients and the variant in exon 18 or the combination of both variants. Other studies in Caucasian population, strong linkage disequilibrium between the exon 16 and exon 18 variants was demonstrated in patients with T2DM but was not shown in the control group [143].

8.1.2. IRS-1gene

The utilization of insulin receptor substrate (IRS)-proteins (IRS-1 and IRS-2) emerged many interactive proteins in the insulin signaling system. This can be amplified or attenuated independently insulin binding and tyrosine kinase activity, providing an extensible mechanism for signal transmission in multiple cellular backgrounds [144]. Patient with T2DM with IRS-1 variants did not differ in their degree of IR compared with patients without known IRS-1 polymorphisms. However, carriers of the codon 972 variant had significantly lower plasma levels of fasting insulin and C-peptide [145, 146]. Many other studies demonstrated several polymorphisms in the IRS-1 gene variant, a Gly-->Arg change at the codon 972 may contribute in impairment of insulin secretion and increased in prevalence among patients with T2DM [146].

8.1.3. PC-1gene

In Swedish and Finnish people, the Q allele of the human glycoprotein PC-1 gene is associated with surrogate measures of IR, but it may not be enough to increase the susceptibility to T2DM. An observation showed there was no difference in the Q allele frequency between the patients with T2DM and control group. There were higher fasting plasma glucose and 2 hours in QK genotype siblings with diabetes compared with carrier of KK genotype. While in sibling with QK genotype and without diabetes have higher fasting plasma glucose and insulin than KK genotype carrier [147].

8.2. Glycogen synthase gene

An Xbal polymorphism has been described in the glycogen synthase gene associated with IR [148]. More features of metabolic syndrome and increased susceptibility to T2DM were described in sibling with rare A2 allele of discordant sib-pair analysis [149]. A set of polymorphic microsatellite markers that span the genome was implemented in genotyping of families with this condition to essence this approach [150].

8.2.1. Calpain 10 (CAPN10) gene

Calpain gene is cytoplasmic cystiene protease requiring calcium ions for activity. CAPN10 gene was proposed as susceptibility locus of T2DM based on the initial report of association between the T2DM and CAPN10 gene [151]. It has been reported of association with T2DM in Pima Indians [152], in African Americans [153] in Mexican Americans [154], in the Botnia area of Finland, German patients [155] and in South Indians [156].

8.2.2. Foxo 1 gene

Insulin signalling downstream of the phosphatidylinositol 3-kinase (PI3K)/Akt pathway is at least in part controls glucose on β-cells mass and function. The activation of Akt is negatively affected the proliferation and metabolism of Foxo transcription factors. The changes in Foxo 1 transcriptional activity are associated with nutritional alteration of β-cells. Glucose-stimulated insulin secretion acts through its own receptor as the predominant mediator of these changes in β-cells [157]. Ghrelin increases pancreatic β-cell proliferation and survival via sequential activation of phosphatidylinositol-3 kinase (PI3K) and Akt ghrelin. It protects pancreatic β-cells from lipotoxicity by inhibiting the nuclear translocation of Foxo1 [158].

8.3. Beta 3-adrenergic receptor gene

The energy balance by increasing in lipolysis and thermogenesis could be regulated by the beta 3-adrenergic receptor (beta 3-AR) gene. The ability to gain weight and the early onset of T2DM are associated with mutation in the beta 3-AR gene (Trp64Arg). But this is not in Dutch population [159]. Many studies in different ethnic groups showed an association of beta3-AR gene polymorphism with IR, obesity and its metabolic disorders such as T2DM, coronary heart disease and hypertension [160].

8.3.1. TCF7L2

The risk alleles of TCF7L2 were associated with enhanced expression of this gene in human islets as well as impaired insulin secretion both in vitro and in vivo. TCF7L2 has also been linked to altered pancreatic islet morphology as exemplified by increased individual islet size and altered α and β cell ratio/distribution within human islets [161]. TCF7L2 encodes the transcription factor TCF4 which is related to Wnt signaling pathway and which plays a critical role in the pathogenesis of T2DM. The risks of alleles in TCF7L2 were associated with hepatic but not peripheral IR and enhanced the rate of hepatic glucose production in human [162]. This is indirectly disturbing beta cells function of the pancreas.

8.3.2. SCL30A8

SCL30A8 encodes the islet specific zinc transporter ZnT-8, which delivers zinc ions from cytoplasm into intracellular insulin-containing granules and is implicated in insulin maturation and/or storage processes in β-cells [163]. The expression level of ZnT-8 was remarkably down regulated in the pancreas of db/db and Akitamice in the early stage of diabetes. Global SCL30A8 knockout mice demonstrated reduced plasma insulin, impaired glucose –stimulated insulin secretion, and markedly reduced islet zinc content [164].

8.4. Others genetic syndromes associated with diabetes

Down syndrome, Klinefelter syndrome, Turner syndrome, Wolfram syndrome, Friedreichataxia, Huntington chorea, Laurence-Moon-Biedlsyndrome, Myotonicdystrophy, Porphyria and Prader-Willi syndrome.

9. Drugs induced hyperglycemia and DM

Many pharmacologic and chemical agents can predispose, induce or precipitate hyperglycemia in normal subjects with high risk of T2DM or patients with IGT and DM. The individual effect of each agent could be weak or strong and subsequently the new glycemic state will be variable from transient to permanent. There are many mechanisms to induce diabetes by interfere with insulin production or secretion (e.g. Beta- Blockers), block insulin action (e.g. Steroids), interfere with both insulin secretion and action (e.g. Thiazides), and finally increase blood glucose using mechanisms independent of insulin's actions (e.g. Nicotinic acid) [165].

Table 2 shows the most common drugs that used in clinical practice with the mechanism of each drug or group.

Drugs	Mechanisms	Notes
Thiazide and thiazide like drugs. Chlorothiazide Chlorothalidone Hydrocholorthiazide Idapamide Methyclothiazide Metolazone	Decreases insulin release by hypokalemia [167,168] and down regulation of PPARγ Receptor.	Avoided in patients with DM and patients at risk of hyperglycemia. Use small dose if requires [167, 168].
*Spironolactone does not cause IGT even at high dosage [167].	In hypertensive elderly on Thiazide but without DM, each 0.5meq/L reduction in serum potassium was associated with 45% higher risk of new DM [169]. Increases aldosterone release and IR [170,171].	Indapamide does not interfere with blood sugar control in T2DM but higher doses that cause potassium loss may cause deterioration. Loop diuretics have been reported to reduce glucose control to a lesser extent than Thiazides [168].
Atypical antipsychotics **High risk** Clozapine Olanzapine **Intermediate risk** Paliperidone Quietiapine Resperidone	Wight gain [172, 173] and adiposity [174] Sympathetic stimulation [175].	Risk of hyperglycemia is more in patients with obesity, age, ethnic status, and certain neuropsychiatric conditions [173].
Low risk Aripiprazole Ziprasidone Unknown Iloperidone	Decrease insulin action [173] and increase IR [176]. Potential Individual Polymorphisms in the leptin gene and leptin receptor gene to antipsychotic induced obesity [177].	
B- blockers Atenolol Metoprolol Propranolol	Increase fasting glucose [178].	The risk of hyperglycemia is increased in patient on B-blocker and thiazide diuretics [180].

Drugs	Mechanisms	Notes
*Carvidolol and nebivolol are not associated with hyperglycemia.	Impair insulin secretion [179]	
Corticosteroids Betamethasone acetate Cortisone Methylprednisolone Hydrocortisone Fludrocortisone Hydrocortisone Triamcinolone Prednisolone Dexamethasone	Decrease in both hepatic and extrahepatic sensitivity to insulin [182].	Identify high risk patient of hyperglycemia.
Oral contraceptive pills	Increase IR [182,183].	Risk of hyperglycemia is increased with higher doses and longer duration therapy.
Megasterol acetate [181].		Monitor the blood glucose to optimize the diabetes therapy by tablets or insulin to avoid short and long term complications of hyperglycemia.
Growth Hormone	Accelerated lipolysis resulting in increased circulating non-esterified fatty acids levels [184,185]. This may contribute to IR, hyperinsulinemia and defective glycogen synthesis [186].	Used as replacement therapy in patients with GH deficiency.
Protease inhibitors Atazanavir, Darunavir Fosamprenavir Indinavir Nelfinavir Ritonivir Saquinavir Tipranivir. Etravirine Maraviroc Raltegravir	Inhibition of GLUT4 Transporter contributes to decrease peripheral insulin sensitivity and induce IR. [187].	Lipodystrophy and Dyslipidaemia are major side effects of this group [188].
Didanosine Nucleoside reverse transcriptase inhibitor	Causes β-cell injury by pancreatitis [189].	Used in treatment of HIV infection. The risk is increased with high dose and in combination with tenofovir [190].
Antibiotics **(Quinolone group)**		

Drugs	Mechanisms	Notes
Gatifloxacin Temafloxacin Levofloxacin	Stimulation of insulin secretion by inhibition of pancreatic beta-cell K(ATP) channels causes hypoglycemia [192]. It may also cause hyperglycemia. [193].	Gatifloxacin was withdrawn from the market because of this effect [193]. Levofloxacin has a small effect. [192].
Rifampicin [191].	Possibly by augmenting intestinal absorption of glucose.	It is an early phase of hyperglycemia and disappeared after few days of treatment. This effect in rat [194].
Tetracyclines Tetracycline chlortetracycline	Causes hyperglycemia.	
\Calcineurin inhibitors Cyclosporine	Impair the function β-cells by impairing insulin gene expression [195-197].	The incidence of new onset DM was 14 to 16% augmented in the first post-transplantation year, declining thereafter to an annual incidence of 4 to 6%, similar to the pre-transplantation baseline rate [205, 206].
Sirolimus Tacrolimus Cyclosporine	Direct β-cells toxicity [198-200]. Decreases in IS [201]. Impair insulin-mediated suppression of hepatic glucose production [202]. May cause ectopic triglyceride deposition, leading to IR [203, 204]. The above aggravated by many modifiable and non-modifiable risk factors [201].	The cumulative incidence of new onset DM was 24% at 3 yr after transplantation [205]. There is a synergetic effect of cyclosporine to induce DM if given with other diabetogenic drug [207].
Thalidomide [208].	Decreases insulin-stimulated peripheral glucose uptake by 31% (increased insulin resistance) Decreases glycogen synthesis by 48%.	Thalidomide, withdrawn for teratogenicity and was reintroduced in 1997 as an immunomodulator to treat erythema nodosum leprosum.
Fish oil or Omega -3 polyunsaturated fatty acids (PUFAs).	PUFAs may affect glucose metabolism through increased IS, but studies to date have been inconclusive [209].	Among all adults who use natural products, more than 37% report taking fish oil or omega-3s. [210].
Interferon α [211].	Risk of hyperglycemia only in patient with chronic hepatitis C infection.	Sustained virological responses reduce the risk of developing glucose abnormalities, especially in patients with normal glucose baseline.

Drugs	Mechanisms	Notes
Ritodrine [212].	Ritodrine induced hypokalemia.	It is selective β2- adrenergic agonist used for premature labour.
Pentamidine [213].	Inappropriate insulin release and toxicity to the islet β-cells. It may cause hypoglycemia, IGT and DM.	It is anti-protozoa agent. These effects worsening with higher doses prolong course and renal impairment.
Statins [214].	Impairing β-cell function and decreasing peripheral insulin sensitivity.	Elderly women and Asians are at particular risk.
Nicotinamide [215].	Enhanced gluconeogenesis.	Hyperglycemia may occur in both normal subjects and in patients with DM.
Diazoxide [216].	Inhibits insulin secretion	Used in treatment of insulinoma.
diphenylhydantoin [217].	Inhibiting apoptosis, increases islet insulin content, accompanied with ameliorated glucose tolerance.	It may be useful in treatment and prevention of DM.
	Inhibits insulin secretion.	Hyperglycemia is more likely to develop in subjects with other risk factors for DM.
L-Asparaginase	Non injury to β-cells [218]. In Rabbits, the anti-tumor enzyme, L-asparaginase, is produced at least in part by the suppression of insulin release [219].	It is transient hyperglycemia that ends following stop the drug.
Vacor Rodenticide poisoning [220].	It has antineoplastic activity and cause pancreatic β-cell damage.	Accidental ingestion by subjects causes severe form of diabetes Ketoacidosis.
Total Parenteral Nutrition	These patients are often critically ill and are administered preparations with high glucose content [221].	It is associated with poor outcome in severely ill patients [221,222].

Table 2. A modified and updated table of mechanisms of drugs induced hyperglycemia [166].

10. Gestational Diabetes Mellitus

Gestational diabetes mellitus (GDM) is a heterogeneous pathogenic condition affecting 2-5% of all pregnant women during pregnancy [223, 224] in other data is 5-6% [225]. GDM and T2DM share a common pathophysiological background, including β-cell dysfunction and IR [226, 227]. In addition, women with GDM are at increased risk of developing T2DM later in life [226]. The pancreatic β- cells failure and impairment is the primary characteristic of GDM. In this group of patients with diabetes, there is a genetic predisposition triggered by increased IR during pregnancy leading to malfunction of the pancreatic β-cells [224]. The clustering of the GDM within family members suggestive of genetic predisposition to the development of this disease. Furthermore, women with MODY gene mutations are reported to have GDM more often [223,224]. In addition, the mutations in other genes include glucokinase (GCK), HLA antigens, insulin receptor (INSR), insulin-like growth factor-2 (IGF2), HNF4A, insulin gene (INS-VNTR), plasminogen activator inhibitor 1 (PAI-1), potassium inwardly rectifying channel subfamily J, member 11 (KCNJ11), hepatocyte nuclear factor-4a (HNF4A) and 1α (HNF1A) [224] suggest the susceptibility to increase the risk of GDM in certain patients.

The stimulators or the inducers of IR and phosphorylate insulin receptor substrate (IRS) proteins are activated in uncontrollable method several kinases, including inhibitor of nuclear factor κB kinase β (IKK β), c-Jun N-terminal kinase (JNK), mammalian target of rapamycin (mTOR), protein kinase C (PKC) and ribosomal S6 protein kinase (S6K). Substance P is a potent cytokine and is considered one of the crucial activators that contribute in the development of IR by impairment of insulin signaling [225]. The genetic variants in TCF7L2 is the strongest gene associated with GDM risk among other minor alleles of rs7903146 (TCF7L2), rs1225 5372 (TCF7L2), rs1799884 (-30G/A, GCK), rs5219 (E23K, KCNJ11), rs7754840 (CDKAL1), rs4402960 (IGF2BP2), rs10830963 (MTNR1B), rs1387153 (MTNR1B) and rs1801278 (Gly972Arg, IRS1) significantly associated with a higher risk of GDM. There are 12 SNPs from 10 genes are associated GDM [228].

The E23K polymorphism of KCNJ11 seems to predispose to GDM in Scandinavian women [226] and the polymorphism of TCF7L2 (rs7903146 C/T) gene, and the G972R polymorphism of the IRS1 gene, seems to predispose to GDM in Greek women [227]. In women of Han nationality in north China, The defect in sulfonylurea receptor-1 (SUR1) gene (cc and AA) may contribute to insulin hypersecretion, which might be the cause of increased body weight and decreased IS and genotype cc of SUR1 is connected with severe type of GDM [229].

In animals but not in human, Galanin inhibits glucose-stimulated insulin release [230]. In the human, the initial postprandial rise of glucose and insulin are suppressed by galanin administration [231]. Galanin and IL-6 were found to be significantly associated with IR markers in GDM, thus may play important roles in the regulation of glucose hemostasis [232]. The higher level of plasma galanin is a novel biomarker for the prediction of GDM [233].

In late pregnancy the relative proinsulin secretion is mainly related to IR and does not necessarily reflect β-cell function. T2DM is not independently associated with hyperproinsulinemia as measured by the proinsulin-to-C-peptide ratio. While, in pregnant women, the increased in IR is associated with decreased proinsulin to C-peptide ratio, independently of glucose tolerance status [234].

The islet amyloid pancreatic polypeptid hypersecretion is characteristic for pregnancy and might partially decrease hyperinsulinemia in pregnancy by inhibiting insulin secretion [235].

The β- cells dysfunction and IR are the core in the pathogenesis of T2DM and both are mediated by Adiponectin. Therefore, in late pregnancy the Adiponectin is an independent factor correlated with β- cells dysfunction [236].

In pregnancy IR and GDM caused by the placental hormones and cytokines such as tumor necrosis factor alpha (TNFα), resisten and leptin. All of these are secreted by placenta independently. The human chorionic somatomammotropin (HCS), cortisol, estrogen, progesterone, and human placental growth hormone (hPGH) are important placental hormones. Severe IR produced by overexpression of hPGH and the increase of the HCS throughout pregnancy stimulates maternal pancreatic insulin release [237].

The fall of IS during pregnancy is counteracted by increase maternal insulin secretion to maintain glucose control [238]. The insufficient insulin secretion to counteract the pregnancy-related decrease in IS is contributing in development of DM [239]. Women at high risk of GDM should have a prior conception plan to prevent DM by normalize body weight, regular physical exercise, reducing excess intake of animal protein and soft drinks, planning of pregnancy in younger ages, avoiding pollutant exposition and smoking cessation [240].

11. Uncommon diseases cause hyperglycemia and DM

11.1. Endocrine diseases

Acromegaly and hypercortisolism are frequently associated with IGT and T2DM. It is a recognized finding of occurrence of secondary T2DM with many hormonal diseases (pituitary, adrenal/or thyroid disease). Patients with Acromegaly have IR, both in the liver and in the periphery displaying hyperinsulinemia and increased glucose turnover in the basal post-absorptive states. There is increase in blood glucose level and free fatty acids due to stimulation of gluconeogenesis and lipolysis. Although, insulin growth factor-1(IGF-1) level is increased but it is unable to counteract IR induced by abnormal excess GH level. On the other hand, IS primarily enhanced in the skeletal muscles by increased IGF-1. The excess of the GH and IGF-1 in patients with Acromegaly could be controlled by somatostatin analogues (SSAs) therapy in most of the patients. On the contrast, the overall glucose tolerance might be complicated by the inhibitory effect of SSAs on pancreatic insulin secretion.

The visceral obesity and IR are induced by hypercortisolemia. It also leads to hyperglycemia and reduced glucose tolerance, determines IR and stimulates hepatic gluconeogenesis and glycogenolysis. The hyperglycemia is due to decreased insulin secretion in patients with neuroendocrine tumors (NETs), patients with pancreatic surgery and in those with pheochro-mocytoma. While in somatostatinoma or gluconoma the hyperglycemia is related to alteration in the counterbalance between these hormones. In the symptomatic treatment of NETs, the SSAs represent a valid therapeutic choice and it may have a significant impact on the preva-lence of glucose metabolism imbalance.

Hyperthyroidism is the principally cause of hyperglycemia among thyroid disorders [241]. IR is associated positively with abnormal increase in the thyroid hormone levels [242]. The uncontrolled diabetes in patient with diabetes developing thyrotoxicosis is related to the stimulation of hepatic glucose production by thyroid hormones acting via a sympathetic pathway from the hypothalamus and FT3 influenced the transcriptional regulators of meta-bolic and mitochondrial genes may contribute to the development of IR. In contrast, hypo-thyroidism is linked to decreased IS. The thyroid hormones have insulin antagonistic effects at the liver that lead to an increase in glucose hepatic output, via an enhanced rate of gluconeogenesis and glycogenolysis. Lipid metabolism (lipogenesis and lipolysis) are stimulated by FT3 further aggravating the dysregulation of liver glucose and lipid metabolism predispose to IR There are several genes are involved in gluconeogenesis, glycogen metabolism, insulin signaling and many hepatic glucogenic enzymes are regulated by thyroid hormones. The thyroid hormones also could cause an increase in hepatic glucose output, through increased hepatic expression of the glucose transporter GLUT2 [243].

11.2. Polycystic ovary syndrome

The features of PCOS are hyperinsulinemia, IR and hyperandrogenesim. The later presented in those patients with hirsutism, acne, irregular periods and reproductive disorders. These features are more marked and severe in obese females and the combination of both (these features with obesity) have a synergistic effect on increased insulin secretion by β-cells and development of compensatory hyperinsulinemia. Subsequently, with the decline of the β-cell compensatory response a relative or absolute insulin secretion and production insufficiency develops which may lead to dysglycemia (IFG, IGT and T2DM). Therefore, it is well-known that PCOS and IR are considered risk factors for GDM [244]. This risk is increased in obese females, presence of family history of T2DM and to the severity of high androgenic activity. Therefore, the dysglycemia could occur in earlier age group than normal population. It could be in the 3rd or 4th decade of life and it is approximately 5 to 10 folds higher than normal population. No doubt, it is higher compared with age and weight matched control age group [245].

11.3. Pancreatic damage or β-cell damage of the pancreas

Chronic alcoholism and tropical calcified pancreatitis are most commonly associated with diabetes [247]. Pancreatic exocrine disease associated with hyperglycemia or DM has a unique clinical and metabolic form. It is painless occasionally and malabsorption occurs after clinical hyperglycemia or DM following failure or impairment of endocrine and exocrine pancreatic function of both α and β cells [246]

11.4. Hereditary hemochromatosis

Iron overload and excessive tissues deposition of iron including the pancreas. It is an autosomal recessive genetic disorder caused by a mutation in the HFE gene located on the short arm of chromosome 6. Approximately 50% of patients diagnosed with hemochromatosis will have either type 1 or T2DM [248].

11.5. Cystic fibrosis

Diabetes Mellitus is the most common morbidity in patients with cystic fibrosis (CF). It occurs in about 20% of adolescent and 40-50% of adults with this disease. CF primarily caused by insulin insufficiency. However, there is a role for IR in acute and chronic stages of this disease due to fluctuation level of insulin. DM has a unique distinct entity in patient with CF because it has mixed features of TIDM and T2DM [249].

Other causes of damage of the pancreas are toxins like alcohol, surgical resection of the pancreas and pancreatic cancer.

11.6. Smoking

There are several studies suggestive of smoking is a risk factor for T2DM, it is an independent and modifiable risk. The early weight gain following smoking cessation is far more beneficial compared with the long term effect of smoking. This weight gain could increase the risk of diabetes [250-252]. Smoking deteriorates glucose metabolism and it is considered a possible a risk factor for development of IR and subsequently T2DM [253]. Smoking is also through a body mass index independent mechanism increasing the risk of T2DM [254, 255]. Pancreatic damage by toxic agents cause insufficient insulin secretion and development of the disease. Tobacco is one of the toxic agent to the human body and organ damage; on the pancreas it is also considered a risk factor of pancreatic cancer and chronic pancreatitis [256].

11.7. Prematurity and birth weight

Hofman PL in 2004 reported an association between low birth weight, commonly a reflection of an adverse in utero environment, and the subsequent development of diseases such as T2DM and hypertension in later life is now generally accepted as is an association between an adverse perinatal environment and a permanent reduction in IS [257, 258].This concept was changed in other report by the evidence has accumulated that small for gestational age children have long-term adult health consequences including obesity, T2DM, hypertension, coronary artery disease and stroke. This increased risk of later adult disease is likely a consequence of an early, persistent reduction in IS [259]. Reduced fetal growth is associated with increased risk of diabetes and suggested a specific association with thinness at birth [260]. Prevalence of T2DM and IGT depended on the synergic effect of thin body size at birth and obesity during adulthood [261]. IGT and T2DM are early signs and indications of growth retardation in early life. The raise in plasma levels of 32-33 split proinsulin is closely related to growth retardation and reflects the β-cells dysfunction [262]. A review and analysis of 14 studies low birth weight (<2,500 g), as compared with a birth weight of >/=2,500 g, was associated with increased risk of T2DM. The risk is the same in high birth weight (>4,000 g), as compared with a birth weight of (</=4,000 g) [263]. The two strongest predictor factors for development of T2DM in adult life are low birth weight and abdominal obesity. The risk of T2DM in Chinese adults is inversely correlated to birth weight. Subjects with high risk of developing hypertension and abdominal obesity are those with the lowest or highest birth weight [264].

12. Conclusion

The evolution of T2DM requires the presence of defects in both insulin secretion and insulin action, and both of these defects can have a genetic and an acquired component. There are many discovered complex alterations in adipose tissue secretion of cytokines, adipokines, and chemokines and immune cell composition observed in adipose tissue-related pathologies such as obesity and IR. The later is a nearly universal finding in patients with established disease. There are many recognized genes involved in β-cell development, function and regulation. These could lead to disorders in insulin secretion, IR and glucose sensing. Physicians should be aware about the potential drugs contribute to the development of hyperglycemia and diabetes. Ladies at high risk of GDM should be identified and screened for diabetes before conception and to be followed after delivery. Early identification and diagnosis of many medical conditions and other risk factors could induce hyperglycemia or precipitate a pre-existing condition of DM.

The above demonstrated a wide range of research in this area that should be encouraged to improve our understanding of the disease. T2DM is a complex interaction between genetics, cytokines, immune cells and tissues during inflammatory responses with obesity, insulin function, IR and β-cells failure. Subsequently this could help in discovery new drugs to treat T2DM that could interfere or stop any stage of these mechanisms at molecular or genetic level.

Author details

Fuad AlSaraj[*]

Address all correspondence to: fuad.alsaraj@mediclinic.ae

Mediclinic Welcare Hospital, Dubai, UAE

References

[1] Defronzo RA. Banting Lecture. From the triumvirate to the ominous octet: a new paradigm for the treatment of type 2 diabetes mellitus. Diabetes 2009; 58 (4):773–795.

[2] Consoli A. Predominant role of gluconeogenesis in increased hepatic glucose production in NIDDM. Diabetes 1989 ;38 (5):550-557.

[3] Consoli A. Role of liver in pathophysiology of NIDDM. Diabetes Care 1992; 15(3): 430-441.

[4] Ramnanan CJ. Physiologic action of glucagon on liver glucose metabolism. Diabetes Obes Metab 2011 ;13 Suppl 1:118-125.

[5] Gerich JE. Control of glycaemia. Baillieres Best Pract Res Clin Endocrinol Metab 1993; 7 (3):551–586.

[6] Porte D Jr, Kahn SE. The key role of islet dysfunction in type II diabetes mellitus. Clin Invest Med 1995; 18 (4):247-254.

[7]   Kahn SE, Porte D Jr. Islet dysfunction in non-insulin-dependent diabetes mellitus. Am J Med. 1988; 85 (5A):4-8.

[8]   Porte D Jr. Banting lecture 1990. Beta-cells in type II diabetes mellitus. Diabetes 1991; 40 (2):166-180.

[9]   Mitrakou A. Contribution of abnormal muscle and liver glucose metabolism to post-prandial hyperglycemia in NIDDM. Diabetes 1990; 39 (11):1381-1390.

[10] Tappy L. Regulation of hepatic glucose production in healthy subjects and patients with non-insulin-dependent diabetes mellitus. Diabete Metab 1995; 21(4):233-240.

[11] Halter JB. Glucose regulation in non-insulin-dependent diabetes mellitus. Interaction between pancreatic islets and the liver. Am J Med 1985; 79 (2B):6-12.

[12] Porte D. β-Cell Dysfunction and Failure in Type 2 Diabetes Potential Mechanisms. Diabetes 2001; 50 (1): S160-S163.

[13] Arthur C. Chapter 78: Insulin, Glucagon, and Diabetes Mellitus. Textbook of Medical Physiology (11th ed.). Philadelphia: Elsevier Saunders 2006. P 963–P968.

[14] Vinay K. Chapter 24: The Endocrine System. Robbins and Cotran Pathologic Basis of Disease (7th ed.). Philadelphia: Elsevier Saunders 2005. P1191–1193.

[15] Cheng K. First phase insulin secretion and type 2 diabetes. Curr Mol Med 2013; 13 (1):126-139.

[16] Byrne MM.Elevated plasma glucose 2 h post challenge predicts defects in β-cell function. Am J Physiol 1996; 270 (4 pt 1): E572-E579.

[17] Gerich JE. Is reduced first-phase insulin release the earliest detectable abnormality in individuals destined to develop type 2 diabetes? Diabetes 2002; 51 (Suppl 1):S117-S121.

[18] Del Prato S. Phasic insulin release and metabolic regulation in type 2 diabetes. Diabetes. 2002 ;51 Suppl 1:S109-S116.

[19] Barg S. A subset of 50 secretory granules in close contact with L-type Ca2+ channels accounts for first-phase insulin secretion in mouse beta-cells. Diabetes 2002; 51 (Suppl 1):S74-S82.

[20] Kühl C. Etiology and pathogenesis of gestational diabetes. Diabetes Care 1998 ;21 Suppl 2:B19-B26.

[21] Nijpels G. Determinants for the progression from impaired glucose tolerance to non-insulin-dependent diabetes mellitus. Eur J Clin Invest 1998 ;28 Suppl 2:8-13.

[22] Abdul-Ghani MA. Contributions of beta-cell dysfunction and insulin resistance to the pathogenesis of impaired glucose tolerance and impaired fasting glucose. Diabetes Care. 2006 ; 29(5):1130-1139.

[23] Magnusson I. Increased rate of gluconeogenesis in type II diabetes mellitus. A ^{13}C nuclear magnetic resonance study. J Clin Invest 1992; 90 (4):1323–1327.

[24] Sesti G. Pathophysiology of insulin resistance. Best Pract Res Clin Endocrinol Metab 2006; 20 (4):665-679.

[25] Ahrén B. Islet adaptation to insulin resistance: mechanisms and implications for intervention. Diabetes Obes Metab 2005; 7 (1):2-8.

[26] Brancati FL. Body weight patterns from 20 to 49 years of age and subsequent risk for diabetes mellitus: the Johns Hopkins Precursors Study. Arch Intern Med 1999; 159 (91):957–963.

[27] Roberts CK. Metabolic Syndrome and Insulin Resistance: Underlying Causes and Modification by Exercise Training. Compr Physio. 2013; 3 (1):1-58.

[28] Petersen KF. Pathogenesis of skeletal muscle insulin resistance in type 2 diabetes mellitus. Am J Cardiol 2002; 90 (5A):11G-18G.

[29] Moller DE. Prevalence of mutations in the insulin receptor gene in subjects with features of the type A syndrome of insulin resistance. Diabetes 1994; 43(2):247-255.

[30] Taylor SI. Insulin resistance associated with androgen excess in women with autoantibodies to the insulin receptor. Ann Intern Med 1982; 97 (6):851-855.

[31] Olshansky SJ. A potential decline in life expectancy in the United States in the 21st century. N Engl J Med 2005; 352 (11): 1138-1145.

[32] Smyth S. Diabetes and obesity: the twin epidemics. Nat Med 2006; 12 (1): 75–80.

[33] Blüher M. Adipose tissue dysfunction in obesity. Exp Clin Endocrinol Diabetes 2009; 117 (6):241-250.

[34] Feng X. PTPRT Regulates High-Fat Diet-Induced Obesity and Insulin Resistance. PLoS One 2014 ;9 (6): e 1100783.

[35] Kahn SE. Mechanisms linking obesity to insulin resistance and type 2 diabetes. Nature 2006; 444(7121):840-846.

[36] Kahn SE. The relative contributions of insulin resistance and beta-cell dysfunction to the pathophysiology of Type 2 diabetes. Diabetologia 2003; 46 (1):3-19.

[37] Meneilly GS. NIDDM in the elderly. Diabetes Care 1996; 19 (12):1320-1325.

[38] Meneilly GS. Metabolic alterations in middle-aged and elderly obese patients with type 2 diabetes. Diabetes Care 1999; 22 (1):112-118.

[39] Ludvik B. Effect of obesity on insulin resistance in normal subjects and patients with NIDDM. Diabetes 1995 ;44 (9):1121-1125.

[40] Boden G. Role of fatty acids in the pathogenesis of insulin resistance and NIDDM. Diabetes. 1997; 46 (1):3-10

[41] Boden G. Effects of free fatty acids (FFA) on glucose metabolism: significance for insulin resistance and type 2 diabetes. Exp Clin Endocrinol Diabetes. 2003; 111 (3): 121-124.

[42] Boden G. Free fatty acids (FFA), a link between obesity and insulin resistance. Front Biosci 1998 15; 3:d169-175.

[43] Boden G. Obesity and Free Fatty Acids (FFA). Endocrinol Metab Clin North Am 2 008; 37 (3): 635–646.

[44] Boden G. Fatty acid-induced inflammation and insulin resistance in skeletal muscle and liver. Curr Diab Rep. 2006; 6(3):177-81.

[45] Shulman G. Cellular mechanisms of insulin resistance. J Clin Invest 2000; 106 (2): 171–176.

[46] Masuzaki H. A transgenic model of visceral obesity and the metabolic syndrome. Science 2001; 294 (5549): 2166–2170.

[47] Rask E. Tissue-specific dysregulation of cortisol metabolism in human obesity. J Clin Endocrinol Metab 2001; 86 (3): 1418–1421.

[48] Paulmyer-Lacroix O. Expression of the mRNA coding for 11β hydroxysteroid dehydrogenase type 1 in adipose tissue from obese patients: An in situ hybridization study. J Clin Endocrinol Metab 2002; 87 (6): 2701–2705.

[49] Hirosumi J. A central role for JNK in obesity and insulin resistance. Nature 2002; 420 (6913): 333–336.

[50] Aguirre V. The c-Jun NH(2)-terminal kinase promotes insulin resistance during association with insulin receptor substrate-1 and phosphorylation of Ser(307). J Biol Chem 2000; 275 (12): 9047– 9054.

[51] Gao Z. Inhibition of insulin sensitivity by free fatty acids requires activation of multiple serine kinases in 3T3-L1 adipocytes. Mol Endocrinol 2004; 18 (8): 2024–2034.

[52] Yuan M. Reversal of obesity- and diet-induced insulin resistance with salicylates or targeted disruption of Ikkbeta. Science 2001; (5539); 293:1673–1677.

[53] Matsuzawa A. ROS-dependent activation of the TRAF6–ASK1–p38 pathway is selectively required for TLR4- mediated innate immunity. Nat Immunol 2005; 6 (6): 587–592.

[54] Shi H. TLR4 links innate immunity and fatty acidinduced insulin resistance. J Clin Invest 2006; 116 (11): 3015–3025.

[55] Suganami T. Role of the Toll-like receptor 4/NF- κB pathway in saturated fatty acid-induced inflammatory changes in the interaction between adipocytes and macrophages. Arterioscler Thromb Vasc Biol 2007; 27 (11): 84–91.

[56] Tobiume K ASK1 is required for sustained activations of JNK/p38 MAP kinases and apoptosis. EMBO Rep 2001; 2 (3): 222–228.

[57] Qatanani M. Mechanisms of obesity-associated insulin resistance: many choices on the menu. Genes Dev 2007; 21 (12): 1443-1455.

[58] Kassem M. Adipose Tissue in Obesity-Related Inflammation and Insulin Resistance: Cells, Cytokines, and Chemokines. ISRN Inflammation 2013; 2013: 139239:1-12.

[59] Piya M. Adipokine inflammation and insulin resistance: the role of glucose, lipids and endotoxin. Journal of Endocrinology 2013; 216 (1): T1–T15.

[60] Cheng KC. Characterization of preptin-induced insulin secretion in pancreatic β-cells. J Endocrinol 2012; 215 (1):43-49.

[61] Buchanan CM. Preptin derived from proinsulin-like growth factor II (proIGF-II) is secreted from pancreatic islet beta-cells and enhances insulin secretion. Biochem J 2001; 360 (pt2):431-439.

[62] Ozkan Y. Acylated and desacylated ghrelin, preptin, leptin, and nesfatin-1 Peptide changes related to the body mass index. Int J Endocrinol 2013; 2013 (236085): 1-7.

[63] Schrauwen P. UCP2 and UCP3 in muscle controlling body metabolism. J Exp Biol. 2002; 205 (pt15):2275-2285.

[64] Zaninovich AA. Role of uncoupling proteins UCP1, UCP2 and UCP3 in energy balance, type 2 diabetes and obesity. Synergism with the thyroid. Medicina (B Aires) 2005; 65 (2):163-169.

[65] Ježek P. Antioxidant and regulatory role of mitochondrial uncoupling protein UCP2 in pancreatic beta-cells. Physiol Res 2014; 63 (Suppl 1):S73-S91.

[66] Pi J. Reactive oxygen species and uncoupling protein 2 in pancreatic β-cell function. Diabetes Obes Metab 2010; 12 (Suppl 2):141-148.

[67] Takata K. Glucose transporters in the transepithelial transport of glucose. J Electron Microsc 1996; 45 (4):275-284.

[68] Scheepers A. The glucose transporter families SGLT and GLUT: molecular basis of normal and aberrant function. JPEN J Parenter Enteral Nutr 2004; 28 (5):364-371.

[69] Watson RT. Intracellular organization of insulin signaling and GLUT4 translocation. Recent Prog Horm Res 2001; 56:175-193.

[70] Haney PM. Intracellular targeting of the insulin-regulatable glucose transporter (GLUT4) is isoform specific and independent of cell type. J Cell Biol 1991;114 (4): 689-699.

[71] Sabino-Silva R. The Na (+)/glucose cotransporters: from genes to therapy. Braz J Med Biol Res 2010; 43(11):1019-1026.

[72] McIntyre EA. Genetics of type 2 diabetes and insulin resistance: knowledge from hu-man studies. Clin Endocrinol (Oxf) 2002; 57 (3):303-311.

[73] Bastian W. Genes with linkage or association with type 2 diabetes mellitus. J Pediatr Endocrinol Metab 2002; 15 (Suppl 1):471-484.

[74] Gibbons Ann. 12th International Congress of Human Genetics. Diabetes Genes De-cline Out of Africa. Science 2011; 334 (6056): 583.

[75] Levine JA. Poverty and Obesity in the U.S. Diabetes 2011, 60: 2667-2668.

[76] Nyamdorj R. BMI compared with central obesity indicators in relation to diabetes and hypertension in Asians. Obesity 2008; 16 (7): 1622-1635.

[77] Boji Huang. Acculturation and Prevalence of Diabetes among Japanese-American Men in Hawaii. Am J Epidemiol 1996; 144:674- 681.

[78] Tuomilehto J. Cardiovascular diseases and diabetes mellitus in Fiji: analysis of mor-tality, morbidity and risk factors. Bull World Health Organ 1984; 62 (1):133-143.

[79] Afable-Munsuz A. Immigrant generation and diabetes risk among Mexican Ameri-cans: the Sacramento area Latino study on aging. Am J Public Health 2014; 104 Suppl 2:S234-S250.

[80] McKeigue PM. Diabetes, hyperinsulinaemia, and coronary risk factors in Banglade-shis in east London. Br Heart J 1988; 60 (5): 390-396.

[81] Enas EA. Coronary heart disease and its risk factors in first-generation immigrant Asian Indians to the United States of America. Indian Heart J 1996; 48 (4): 343-353.

[82] Van Dam RM. The epidemiology of lifestyle and risk for type 2 diabetes. Eur J Epide-miol 2003; 18 (12): 1115-1125.

[83] Shaw J. Epidemiology and prevention of type 2 diabetes and the metabolic syn-drome. MJA 2003; 179 (7): 379-383.

[84] Zimmett P. Global and societal implication of the diabetes epidemic. Nature 2001; 414 (6865): 782-787.

[85] Lean ME. Obesity: burdens of illness and strategies for prevention or management. Drugs Today (Barc) 2000; 36 (11): 773-784.

[86] Fagot-Campagna A. Type 2 diabetes among North American children and adoles-cents: an epidemiologic review and a public health perspective. J Pediatr 2000; 136 (5): 664-672.

[87] Sinha R. Prevalence of impaired glucose tolerance among children and adolescents with marked obesity. N Engl J Med 2002;346 (11): 802-810.

[88] Hu FB. Sedentary lifestyle and risk of obesity and type 2 diabetes. Lipids 2003; 38 (2): 103-108.

[89] Pan XR. Effects of diet and exercise in preventing NIDDM in people with impaired glucose tolerance. The Da Qing IGT and Diabetes Study. Diabetes Care 1997; 20 (4): 537-544.

[90] Tuomilehto J. Prevention of type 2 diabetes mellitus by changes in lifestyle among subjects with impaired glucose tolerance. N Engl J Med 2001; 344 (18): 1343-1350.

[91] Knowler WC. Reduction in the Incidence of Type 2 Diabetes with Lifestyle Intervention or Metformin. N Engl J Med 2002; 346 (6):393-403.

[92] Xue Sun. Genetics of Type 2 Diabetes: Insights into the Pathogenesis and Its Clinical Application. BioMed Research International 2014; 2014 (926713): 1-15.

[93] Steinthorsdottir V. A variant in CDKAL1 influences insulin response and risk of type 2 diabetes. Nature Genetics 2007; 39 (6): 770-775.

[94] Voight BF. Twelve type 2 diabetes susceptibility loci identified through large-scale association analysis. Nature Genetics 2010; 42 (7): 579–589.

[95] Silander K. Genetic variation near the hepatocyte nuclear factor-4α gene predicts susceptibility to type 2 diabetes. Diabetes 2004; 53 (4): 1141–1149.

[96] Lyssenko V. Common variant in MTNR1B associated with increased risk of type 2 diabetes and impaired early insulin secretion. Nature 2009; 41(1): 82-88.

[97] Nielsen T. Type 2 diabetes risk allele near CENTD2 is associated with decreased glucose-stimulated insulin release. Diabetologia 2011; 54 (5):1052–1056.

[98] Boesgaard TW. Variant near ADAMTS9 known to associate with type 2 diabetes is related to insulin resistance in offspring of type 2 diabetes patients— EUGENE2 study. PLoS ONE 2009; 4: (9): e7236.

[99] Anand A. In vivo modulation of Hmgic reduces obesity. Nature Genetics 2000; 24 (4): 377–380.

[100] Rung J. Genetic variant near IRS1 is associated with type 2 diabetes, insulin resistance and hyperinsulinemia. Nature Genetics 2009; 41(10): 1110–1115.

[101] Binh T. Association of the common FTO-rs9939609 polymorphism with type 2 diabetes, independent of obesity-related traits in a Vietnamese population. Gene 2013; 513 (1): 31–35.

[102] Xi B. Common polymorphism near the MC4R gene is associated with type 2 diabetes: data fromameta-analysis of 123, 373 individuals. Diabetologia 2012; 55 (10): 2660–2666.

[103] Barnett AH. Diabetes in identical twins: A study of 200 pairs. Diabetologia 1981; 20 (2): 87–93.

[104] Committee on Diabetic Twins, Japan Diabetes Society. Diabetes mellitus in twins: a cooperative study in Japan. Committee on Diabetic Twins, Japan Diabetes Society. Diabetes Res Clin Pract 1988 14; 5 (4):271-280.

[105] Matsuda A. Relationship between obesity and concordance rate for type 2 (non-insulin-dependent) diabetes mellitus among twins. Diabetes Res Clin Pract 1994; 26 (2): 137-143.

[106] Kobberling J., Tillil H. Empirical risk figures for first-degree relatives of non-insulin dependent diabetics. In The Genetics of Diabetes Mellitus. (ed J. Kobberling, R Tattersall 1982. p201–p209.

[107] Eriksson J. Early metabolic defects in persons at increased risk for non- insulin-dependent diabetes mellitus. N Engl J Med 1989; 321 6): 337–343.

[108] Humphriss DB. Multiple metabolic abnormalities in normal glucose tolerant relatives of NIDDM families. Diabetologia 1997; 40 (10):1185–1190.

[109] Lillioja S. In vivo insulin action is familial characteristic in nondiabetic Pima Indians. Diabetes 1987; 36 (11):1329–1335.

[110] Martin BC. Familial clustering of insulin sensitivity. Diabetes 1992; 41 (7): 850–854.

[111] Henry RR. Insulin action and glucose metabolism in nondiabetic control and NIDDM subjects. Comparison using human skeletal muscle cell cultures. Diabetes 1995; 44 (8): 936–946.

[112] Jackson S. Decreased insulin responsiveness of glucose uptake in cultured human skeletal muscle cells from insulin-resistant nondiabetic relatives of type 2 diabetic families. Diabetes 2000; 49 (7):1169–1177.

[113] DeFronzo RA. Insulin resistance. A multifaceted syndrome responsible for NIDDM, obesity, hypertension, dyslipidemia, and atherosclerotic cardiovascular disease. Diabetes Care 1991; 14 (3):173–194.

[114] Frayling TM. Beta-cell genes and diabetes: molecular and clinical characterization of mutations in transcription factors. Diabetes 2001; 50 (Suppl 1):S94-S100.

[115] Gardner DS. Clinical features and treatment of maturity onset diabetes of the young (MODY). Diabetes Metab Syndr Obes 2012; 5: 101–108.

[116] Shepherd M. Predictive genetic testing in maturity-onset diabetes of the young (MODY) Diabet Med 2001; 18 (5):417–421.

[117] Froguel P. Close linkage of glucokinase locus on chromosome 7p to early-onset non-insulin-dependent diabetes mellitus. Nature 1992; 356 (6365):162 –164.

[118] Hattersley AT. Linkage of type 2 diabetes to the glucokinase gene. Lancet 1992; 339 (8805):1307–1310.

[119] Yamagata K. Mutations in the hepatocyte nuclear factor-4α gene in maturity-onset diabetes of the young (MODY1). Nature 1996; 384 (6608):458 –460.

[120] Yamagata K. Mutations in the hepatocyte nuclear factor-1α gene in maturity-onset diabetes of the young (MODY3). Nature 1996; 384 (6608):455–458.

[121] Alessandro D. Recent advances in the genetics of maturity onset diabetes of the young and other forms of autosomal dominant diabetes. Curr Opin Endocrinol & Diabetes 2000; 7 (4):203–210.

[122] McDonald TJ. Maturity onset diabetes of the young: identification and diagnosis. Ann Clin Biochem 2013; 50 (pt5):403-415.

[123] Stoffers DA. Early-onset type-II diabetes mellitus (MODY4) linked to IPF1. Nat Genet 1997; 17 (2):138-139.

[124] Horikawa Y. Mutation in hepatocyte nuclear factor-1 beta gene (TCF2) associated with MODY. Nat Genet 1997; 17 (4):384 –385.

[125] Malecki MT. Mutations in NEUROD1 are associated with the development of type 2 diabetes mellitus. Nat Genet 1999; 23 (3):323-328.

[126] Rochelle Naylor. Who should have genetic testing for maturity-onset diabetes of the young?. Clinical Endocrinology (Oxf) 2011; 75 (4): 422–426.

[127] Timsit J. Diagnosis and management of maturity-onset diabetes of the young. Treat Endocrinol 2005; 4 (1):9-18.

[128] GotoY. A mutation in the tRNA (Leu) (UUR) gene associated with the MELAS subgroup of mitochondrial encephalomyopathies. Nature1990; 348 (6302): 651–653.

[129] Vanden Ouweland JM. Mutation in mitochondrial tRNA (Leu) (UUR) gene in a large pedigree with maternally transmitted type II diabetes mellitus and deafness. Nat Genet 1992; 1 (5): 368–371.

[130] Maassen JA. Maternally inherited diabetes and deafness: a new diabetes subtype. Diabetologia 1996; 39 (4): 375–82.

[131] Vionnet N. Prevalence of mitochondrial gene mutations in families with diabetes mellitus. Lancet 1993; 342 (8884):1429–1430.

[132] Newkirk JE. Maternally inherited diabetes and deafness: prevalence in a hospital diabetic population. Diabet Med 1997; 14 (6): 457–460.

[133] Daly MJ. High resolution haplotype structure in the human genome. Nat Genet 2001; 29 (2):229-232.

[134] Krook A. Mutant insulin receptors in syndromes of insulin resistance. Clin Endocrinolo Metab 1996; 10 (1): 97–122.

[135] Whitehead JP. Molecular scanning of the insulin receptor substrate 1 gene in subjects with severe insulin resistance: detection and functional analysis of a naturally occurring mutation in a YMXM motif. Diabetes 1998; 47 (5): 837–838.

[136] Whitehead JP. Multiple molecular mechanisms of insulin receptor dysfunction in a patient with Donohue syndrome. Diabetes 1998; 47 (8):1362–1364.

[137] Hegele RA. Familial partial lipodystrophy: a monogenic form of the insulin resistance syndrome. Mole Genet Metab 2000; 71(4): 539–544.

[138] Shackleton S. LMNA, encoding lamin A/C, is mutated in partial lipodystrophy. Nat Genet 2000; 24 (2): 153–156.

[139] Hegele RA. Premature atherosclerosis associated with monogenic insulin resistancze. Circulation 2001; 103 (18): 2225–2229.

[140] Martin G. Coordinate regulation of the expression of the fatty acid transport protein and acyl-CoA synthetase genes by PPARalpha and PPARgamma activators. J Biol Chem 1997; 272(45):28210-28217.

[141] Barroso I. Dominant negative mutations in human PPARgamma associated with severe insulin resistance, diabetes mellitus and hypertension. Nature 1999; 402 (6764): 880–883.

[142] Huxtable SJ. Analysis of parent–offspring trios provides evidence for linkage and association between the insulin gene and type 2 diabetes mediated exclusively through paternally transmitted class III variable number tandem repeat alleles. Diabetes 2000; 49 (1): 126–130.

[143] Hart LM. Variants in the sulphonylurea receptor gene: association of the exon 16-3t variant with Type II diabetes mellitus in Dutch Caucasians. Diabetologia 1999; 42 (5): 617-620.

[144] White MF. The insulin signalling system and the IRS proteins. Dibetologia 1997; 40 (Suppl 2): S2-17.

[145] Almind K. Aminoacid polymorphisms of insulin receptor substrate-1 in non-insulin-dependent diabetes mellitus. Lancet 1993; 342 (8875): 828–832.

[146] Porzio O. The Gly972 → Arg amino acid polymorphism in IRS-1 impairs insulin secretion in pancreatic beta cells. J Clin Invest 1999; 104 (3): 357–364.

[147] Gu HF. Association between the human glycoprotein PC-1 gene and elevated glucose and insulin levels in a paired-sibling analysis. Diabetes 2000; 49 (9):1601–1603.

[148] Groop LC. Association between polymorphism of the glycogen synthase gene and non-insulin-dependent diabetes mellitus. N Eng J Med 1993; 328 (1):10–14.

[149] Orho-Melander M. A paired-sibling analysis of the XbaI polymorphism in the muscle glycogen synthase gene. Diabetologia 1999; 42 (9):1138–1145.

[150] McIntyre EA. Genetics of type 2 diabetes and insulin resistance: knowledge from hu-
       man studies. Clin Endocrinol (Oxf) 2002; 57 (3):303-311.

[151] Horikawa Y. Genetic variation in the calapin 10 gene (CAPN10) is associated with
       type 2 diabetes mellitus. Nat Genet 2000; 26 (2): 163-175.

[152] Baier LJ. A calpain- 10 gene polymorphysim is associated with reduced muscle
       mRNA levels and insulin resistance. J Clin Invest 2000; 106 (7): R69-73.

[153] Garant MJ. SNP43 of CAPN10 and the risk of type 2 diabetes in African-Americans:
       the Atherosclerosis Risk in Communities Study. Diabetes 2002; 51(1):231–237.

[154] del Bosque-Plata L. Association of the calpain-10 gene with type 2 diabetes mellitus
       in a Mexican population. Mol Genet Metab 2004; 81(2):122-126.

[155] Fingerlin TE. Variation in three single nucleotide polymorphisms in the calpain-10
       gene not associated with type 2 diabetes in a large Finnish cohort. Diabetes 2002; 51
       (5):1644-1648.

[156] Cassell PG. Haplotype combinations of calpain 10 gene polymorphisms associate
       with increased risk of impaired glucose tolerance and type 2 diabetes in South Indi-
       ans. Diabetes 2002; 51(5):1622–1628.

[157] Martinez SC. Glucose regulates Foxo1 through insulin receptor signaling in the pan-
       creatic islet beta-cell. Diabetes 2006; 55 (6):1581-1591.

[158] Wang W. Inhibition of Foxo1 mediates protective effects of ghrelin against lipotoxici-
       ty in MIN6 pancreatic beta-cells. Peptides 2010; 31(1):307-314.

[159] Oeveren van-Dybicz AM. Beta 3-adrenergic receptor gene polymorphism and type 2
       diabetes in a Caucasian population. Diabetes Obes and Metab 2001; 3 (1):47-51.

[160] Babol K. Beta3-adrenergic receptor. Postepy Biochem 2005; 51(1):80-87.

[161] Le Bacquer O. TCF7L2 rs7903146 impairs islet function and morphology in nondia-
       betic individuals. Diabetologia 2012; 55 (10): 2677–2681.

[162] Lyssenko V. Mechanisms by which common variants in the TCF7L2 gene increase
       risk of type 2 diabetes. The Journal of Clinical Investigation 2007; 117 (8):2155–2163.

[163] Chimienti F. ZnT-8, a pancreatic β-cell specific zinc transporter. Biometals 2005; 18
       (4): 313–317.

[164] Pound LD. Deletion of the mouse Slc30a8 gene encoding zinc transporter-8 results in
       impaired insulin secretion. Biochemical Journal 2009; 421 (3): 371–376.

[165] Lohani Gaya. Drug- induced diabetes. Medicine Update 2010; 20 (72): 70-73.

[166] Abdur Rehman. Drug-Induced Glucose Alterations Part 2: Drug-Induced Hypergly-
       cemia. Diabetes Spectrum 2011; 24 (4):234-238.

[167] Ramsay LE. Diabetes, impaired glucose tolerance and insulin resistance with diuretics. Eur Heart J 1992; 13 (Suppl G):68-71.

[168] O'Byrne S. Effects of drugs on glucose tolerance in non-insulin-dependent diabetics (Part I). Drugs 1990; 40 (1):6-18.

[169] Shafi T. Changes in serum potassium mediate thiazide-induced diabetes. Hypertension 2008; 52 (6):1022-1029.

[170] Carter B. Thiazide-induced dysglycemia: call for research from a working group from the National Heart, Lung, and Blood Institute. Hypertension 2008; 52 (1):30–36.

[171] Tham DM. Angtiotensin II is associated with activation of NF- kB-mediated genes and downregulation of PPARS. Physiol Genomics 2002; 11(1):21–30.

[172] Henderson DC. Clozapine, diabetes mellitus, weight gain, and lipid abnormalities: A five-year naturalistic study. Am J Psychiatry. 2000; 157 (6):975-981.

[173] Haupt DW. Hyperglycemia and antipsychotic medications. J Clin Psychiatry 2001; 62 (Suppl 27):15-26.

[174] Newcomer JW. Second-generation (atypical) antipsychotics and metabolic effects: a comprehensive literature review. CNS Drugs 2005; 19 (Suppl 1):1-93.

[175] Savoy YE. Differential effects of various typical and atypical antipsychotics on plasma glucose and insulin levels in the mouse: evidence for the involvement of sympathetic regulation. Schizophr Bull 2010; 36 (2):410–418.

[176] Leung JY. Cardiovascular side-effects of antipsychotic drugs: the role of the autonomic nervous system. Pharmacol Ther 2012; 135(2):113-122.

[177] Lee AK. Pharmacogenetics of leptin in antipsychotic-associated weight gain and obesity-related complications. Pharmacogenomics 2011; 12 (7):999-1016.

[178] Luna B. Drug-induced hyperglycemia. JAMA 2001; 286 (16):1945–1948.

[179] Greiss TW. Hypertension and antihypertensive therapy as risk factors for type 2 diabetes mellitus. N Engl J Med 2000; 342 (3) :905.

[180] Ferner RE. Drug-induced diabetes. Baillieres Clin Endocrinol Metab 1992;6 (4):849-66.

[181] Henry K. Diabetes mellitus induced by megestrol acetate in a patient with AIDS and cachexia. Ann Intern Med 1992 1; 116(1):53-54.

[182] Rizza RA. Cortisol-induced insulin resistance in man: impaired suppression of glucose production and stimulation of glucose utilization due to a postreceptor detect of insulin action. J Clin Endocrinol Metab 1982; 54 (1): 131-138.

[183] Paquot N. Effects of glucocorticoids and sympathomimetic agents on basal and insulin-stimulated glucose metabolism. Clin Physiol 1995; 15(3):231-240.

[184] Bak JF. Effects of growth hormone on fuel utilization and muscle glycogen synthase activity in normal humans. Am J Physiol 1991; 260 (5pt1):E736-E742.

[185] Sherwin RS. Effect of growth hormone on oral glucose tolerance and circulating metabolic fuels in man. Diabetologia 1983; 24 (3):155-161.

[186] Manthinda H. Growth Hormone-Induced Insulin Resistance and Its Relationship to Lipid Availability in the Rat. Diabetes 1996; 45 (4): 415-421.

[187] Joseph C. HIV Protease Inhibitors Acutely Impair Glucose-Stimulated Insulin Release. Diabetes 2003; 52 (7): 1695-1700.

[188] Calvo M. Update on metabolic issues in HIV patients. Curr Opin HIV AIDS 2014; 9 (4):332-339.

[189] Munshi M. Hyperosmolar nonketotic diabetic syndrome following treatment of human deficiency virus infection with didanosine. Diabetes Care 1994; 17(4): 316.

[190] Pecora F. Effect of tenofovir on didanosine absorption in patients with HIV. Ann Pharmacother 2003; 37 (9): 1325-1328.

[191] Takasu N. Rifampicin-induced early phase hyperglycemia in humans. Am Rev Respir Dis 1982; 125 (1):23-27.

[192] Saraya A. Effects of fluoroquinolones on insulin secretion and beta-cell ATP-sensitive K+ channels. Eur J Pharmacol 2004; 497 (1):111-117.

[193] Aspinall SL. Severe Dysglycemia with the Fluoroquinolones: A Class Effect? Clin Infect Dis 2009; 49 (3): 402-408.

[194] Storozhuk PG. Effect of certain antibiotics of tetracycline series on the level of blood sugar and the role of insulin in the mechanism of its regulation. Probl Endokrinol (Mosk) 1976 ;22 (6):106-110.

[195] Redmon JB. Effects of tacrolimus (FK506) on human insulin gene expression, insulin mRNA levels, and insulin secretion in HIT-T15 cells. J Clin Invest 1996; 98 (12): 2786–2793.

[196] Herold KC. Inhibition of glucose-stimulated insulin release from beta TC3 cells and rodent islets by an analog of FK506. Transplantation 1993; 55(1): 186–192.

[197] Hahn HJ.Reversibility of the acute toxic effect of cyclosporine A on pancreatic B cells of Wistar rats. Diabetologia 1986; 29(8): 489–494.

[198] Kwon G. Glucose-stimulated DNA synthesis through mammalian target of rapamycin (mTOR) is regulated by KATP channels: Effects on cell cycle progression in rodent islets. J Biol Chem 2006; 281(6): 3261–3267.

[199] Kwon G. Signaling elements involved in the metabolic regulation of mTOR by nutrients, incretins, and growth factors in islets. Diabetes 2004; 53(Suppl 3): S225–S232.

[200] Bussiere CT. The impact of the mTOR inhibitor sirolimus on the proliferation and function of pancreatic islets and ductal cells. Diabetologia 2006; 49 (10): 2341–2349.

[201] Micheal F. Transplant-Associated Hyperglycemia: A New Look at an old problem. Clin J Am Soc Nephrol 2007; 2(2):343-355.

[202] Kasiske BL. Diabetes mellitus after kidney transplantation in the United States. Am J Transplant 2003; 3 (2) 178–185.

[203] Woodward RS. Incidence and cost of new onset diabetes mellitus among US wait-listed and transplanted renal allograft recipients. Am J Transplant 2003; 3 (5): 590–598.

[204] Syed NA. Reciprocal regulation of glycogen phosphorylase and glycogen synthase by insulin involving phosphatidylinositol-3 kinase and protein phosphatase- 1 in HepG2 cells. Mol Cell Biochem 2000; 211(1-2): 123–136.

[205] Mittelman SD. Inhibition of lipolysis causes suppression of endogenous glucose production independent of changes in insulin. Am J Physiol Endocrinol Metab 2000; 279 (3): E630–E637.

[206] Lewis GF. Disordered fat storage and mobilization in the pathogenesis of insulin resistance and type 2 diabetes. Endocr Rev 2002; 23(2): 201–229.

[207] Ost L. impaired glucose tolerance in cyclosporine-prednisone treated renal graft recipients. Transplant 1988; 46 (3): 370-372.

[208] Wilson JS. Congenital deformities and insulin antagonism. Lancet 1996; 2 (7470): 940–941.

[209] Akinkuolie AO. Omega-3 polyunsaturated fatty acid and insulin sensitivity: a meta-analysis of randomized controlled trials. Clin Nutr 2011; 30 (6):702-707.

[210] Barnes PM. Complementary and alternative medicine use among adults and children: United States, 2007. Natl Health Stat Report 2008; 10 (12):1-23.

[211] Zhang W. Effects of interferon-alpha treatment on the incidence of hyperglycemia in chronic hepatitis C patients: a systematic review and meta-analysis. PLoS One 2012 (6); 7:e39272.

[212] Cano A. Metabolic disturbances during intravenous use of ritodrine: increased insulin levels and hypokalemia. Obstet Gynecol 1985; 65 (3):356-360.

[213] Roger A. Pentamidine-Induced Derangements of Glucose Homeostasis. Diabetes Care 1995; 18 (1): 49-55.

[214] Goldstein MR. Do statins cause diabetes? Curr Diab Rep 2013; 13 (3):381-390.

[215] Henkin Y. Niacin revisited: clinical observations on an important but underutilized drug. Am J Med 1991; 91(3):239-246.

[216] Huang Q. Diazoxide prevents diabetes through inhibiting pancreatic beta-cells from apoptosis via Bcl-2/Bax rate and p38-beta mitogen-activated protein kinase. Endocrinology 2007; 148 (1): 81–91.

[217] Fariss BL. Diphenylhydantoin-induced hyperglycemia and impaired insulin release. Effect of dosage. Diabetes. 1971;20 (3):177-181.

[218] Gailau S. Diabetes in patients treated with asparaginase. Clin Pharmacol Ther 1971; 12(3): 487.

[219] Lavine RL. E.coli L-asparaginase and insulin release in vitro. Metabolism. 1982; 31(10):1009-1013.

[220] Leona VM. Diabetes Mellitus and Autonomic Dysfunction After Vacor Rodenticide Ingestion. Diabetes Care 1978; 1(2):73-76.

[221] Cheung NW. Hyperglycemia Is Associated With Adverse Outcomes in Patients Receiving Total Parenteral Nutrition. Diabetes Care 2005; 28 (10): 267-271.

[222] Francisco J. Hyperglycemia During Total Parenteral Nutrition An important marker of poor outcome and mortality in hospitalized patients. Diabetes Care 2010; 33 (4): 739–741.

[223] Shaat N. Genetics of gestational diabetes mellitus. Curr Med Chem 2007; 14 (5): 569-583.

[224] Lambrinoudaki I. Genetics in gestational diabetes mellitus: association with incidence, severity, pregnancy outcome and response to treatment. Curr Diabetes Rev 2010; 6 (6): 393-399.

[225] Patro-Malysza J. The Impact of Substance P on the Pathogenesis of Insulin Resistance Leading to Gestational Diabetes. Curr Pharm Biotechnol 2014; 15(1):32-37.

[226] Shaat N. Association of the E23K polymorphism in the KCNJ11 gene with gestational diabetes mellitus. Diabetologia 2005; 48 (12):2544-2551.

[227] Pappa KI. Gestational diabetes mellitus shares polymorphisms of genes associated with insulin resistance and type 2 diabetes in the Greek population. Gynecol Endocrinol 2011; 27 (4):267-272.

[228] Zhang C. Genetic variants and the risk of gestational diabetes mellitus: a systematic review. Hum Reprod Update 2013; 19 (4):376-390.

[229] Niu XM. Study on association between gestational diabetes mellitus and sulfonylurea receptor-1 gene polymorphism. Zhonghua Fu Chan Ke Za Zhi 2005; 40 (3):159-163.

[230] Holst JJ. On the effects of human galanin in man. Diabetologia 1993; 36 (7):653–657.

[231] Bauer FE. Inhibitory effect of galanin on postprandial gastrointestinal motility and gut hormone release in humans. Gastroenterology 1989; 97 (2):260–264.

[232] Nergiz S. Circulating galanin and IL-6 concentrations in gestational diabetes mellitus. Gynecol Endocrinol 2014; 30 (3):236-240.

[233] Zhang Z. Endogenous galanin as a novel biomarker to predict gestational diabetes mellitus. Peptides 2014; 54:186-189.

[234] Retnakaran R. The impact of insulin resistance on proinsulin secretion in pregnancy: hyperproinsulinemia is not feature of gestational diabetes. Diabetes Care 2005; 28 (11):2710-2715.

[235] Kautzky-Willer A. Elevated islet amyloid pancreatic polypeptide and proinsulin in lean gestational diabetes. Diabetes 1997; 46 (4):607-614.

[236] Retnakaran R. Adiponectin and beta cell dysfunction in gestational diabetes: pathophysiological implications. Diabetologia 2005; 48 (5):993-1001.

[237] Metzger BE. Summary and recommendations of the Fifth International Workshop-Conference on Gestational Diabetes Mellitus. Diabetes Care 2007; 30 (suppl 2):S251–S260.

[238] Sullivan B. Gestational diabetes. J Am Pharm Assoc 1998; 38 (3):364-371.

[239] Vambergue A. Pathophysiology of gestational diabetes. J Gynecol Obstet Biol Reprod (Paris) 2002; 31(6 suppl):4S3-4S10.

[240] Kleinwechter H. Predisposition and phenotypes of gestational diabetes. Dtsch Med Wochenschr 2014; 139 (21):1123-1126.

[241] Resmini E. Secondary diabetes associated with principal endocrinopathies: the impact of new treatment modalities. Acta Diabetol 2009; 46 (2):85-95.

[242] Lambadiari V. Thyroid hormones are positively associated with insulin resistance early in the development of type 2 diabetes. Endocrine 2011; 39 (1):28-32.

[243] Brenta G. Why Can Insulin Resistance Be a Natural Consequence of Thyroid Dysfunction? Journal of Thyroid Reserch 2011; 2011: 152850, 9 pages.

[244] De Leo V. Polycystic ovary syndrome and type 2 diabetes mellitus. Minerva Ginecol 2004; 56 (1): 53-62.

[245] Pelusi B. Type 2 diabetes and the polycystic ovary syndrome. Minerva Ginecol 2004; 56 (1):41-51.

[246] Sjoberg RJ. Pancreatic diabetes mellitus. Diabetes Care 1989; 12 (10):715-724.

[247] Choudhuri G. Pancreatic diabetes. Trop Gastroenterol 2009; 30 (2):71-75.

[248] Richard JS. Case Study: Screening and Treatment of Pre-Diabetes in Primary Care. Clinical Diabetes 2004; 22 (2): 98-104.

[249] Moran A. Clinical Care Guidelines for Cystic Fibrosis–Related Diabetes. A position statement of the American Diabetes Association and a clinical practice guideline of

the Cystic Fibrosis Foundation, endorsed by the Pediatric Endocrine Society. Diabetes Care 2010; 33 (12): 2697–2708.

[250] Yeh HC. Smoking cessation and risk for type 2 diabetes mellitus. A cohort study Annals of Internal Medicine 2010; 152(1): 10-17.

[251] Rimm EB. Prospective study of cigarette smoking, alcohol use, and the risk of diabetes in men. BMJ1995; 310 (6979): 555–559.

[252] Radzeviciene L. Smoking habits and the risk of type 2 diabetes: a case control study. Diabetes and Metabolism 2009; 35 (3):192-197.

[253] Fagard RH. Smoking and diabetes – the double health hazard. Primary Care Diabetes 2009; 3 (4): 205-209.

[254] Cullen MW. No interaction of body mass index and smoking on diabetes mellitus risk in elderly women. Preventative Medicine 2009; 48(1): 74-78.

[255] Nagaya T. Heavy smoking raises risk for type 2 diabetes milletus in obese men; but, light smoking reduces the risk in lean men: a follow up study in Japan. Annals of Epidemiology 2008; 18(2): 113-118.

[256] Lynch SM. Cigarette smoking and pancreatic cancer: a pooled analysis from the pancreatic cancer cohort consortium. American Journal of Epidemiology 2009; 170(4): 403-413.

[257] Hofman PL. Premature birth and later insulin resistance. N Engl J Med 2004; 351(21): 2179-2186.

[258] Hofman PL. The metabolic consequences of prematurity. Growth Horm IGF Res. 2004;14 (Suppl A):S136-S139.

[259] Hofman PL. Insulin sensitivity in people born pre-term, with low or very low birth weight and small for gestational age. J Endocrinol Invest 2006; 29 (1 Suppl):2-8.

[260] Lithell HO. Relation of size at birth to non-insulin dependent diabetes and insulin concentrations in men aged 50-60 years. BMJ 1996; 312 (7028):406-410.

[261] Mi J. Association of body size at birth with impaired glucose tolerance during their adulthood for men and women aged 41 to 47 years in Beijing of China. Zhonghua Yu Fang Yi Xue Za Zhi 1999; 33 (4):209-213.

[262] Hales CN. Fetal and infant growth and impaired glucose tolerance at age 64. BMJ. 1991; 303 (6809):1019-1022.

[263] Harder T. Birth weight and subsequent risk of type 2 diabetes: a meta-analysis. Am J Epidemiol 2007; 165 (8):849-857.

[264] Tian JY. Birth weight and risk of type 2 diabetes, abdominal obesity and hypertension among Chinese adults. Eur J Endocrinol 2006; 155(4):601-607.

Complication of Type 1 Diabetes in Craniofacial and Dental Hard Tissue

Ippei Watari, Mona Aly Abbassy, Katarzyna Anna Podyma-Inoue and Takashi Ono

Abstract

Diabetes mellitus (DM) is a chronic systemic disease arisen under the conditions when the body cannot produce enough insulin or cannot use it effectively. Type 1 diabetes is caused by an autoimmune reaction, where the body's defense system attacks the insulin-producing β-cells in the pancreas. Type 1 diabetes incidence has been rising all over the world, especially under the age of 15 years. There are strong premonitions of geographic difference; however, the overall annual increase in a number of affected population is estimated to be approximately 3%.

Under these circumstances, detailed understanding of the influence of type 1 diabetes on various organs is integrant. The systematic diseases have been seen to have a considerable effect on bone. As such, diabetes also exerts some degree of influence on bone in general. Hyperglycemia or impaired glucose metabolism has a number of detrimental effects on bone metabolism; for example, it is well documented that bone mass decreases and rate of bone fracture risk increases in type 1 diabetes patients. Nonetheless, there are few reports describing the influence of type 1 diabetes on hard tissue in craniofacial region.

From a dental clinical perspective, uncontrolled diabetic condition is thought to be one of the main causative factors of increased risk of inflammation and dental caries that lead to tooth loss and may also increase the risk of cardiovascular disease or preterm birth. However, there are only few reports focusing on type 1 diabetes complication in oral and maxillofacial region. Thus, in this chapter, we summarize the complication of type 1 diabetes in craniofacial hard tissue. Based on our previous data, type 1 diabetes lead to the retardant effects in cranium, mandible, and teeth during early growth period. This information is of critical importance not only for the better understanding of the type 1 diabetes complication in jaw or teeth but also for the development of efficient treatment and prevention of oral diseases in type 1 diabetes patients.

Keywords: Craniofacial complex, growth, type I diabetes, gestational diabetes

1. Introduction

Type 1 diabetes is a chronic and a complex autoimmune disease arisen primarily due to β-cell destruction. Historically, type 1 diabetes was considered as a disorder in children and adolescents, but now it is known that symptomatic onset of type 1 diabetes may occur at any age. Three major symptoms, polydipsia, polyphagia, and polyuria along with overt hyperglycemia, are a diagnostic hallmark in young type 1 diabetes patients. Exogenous insulin replacement is needed immediately after the onset of type 1 diabetes and should be kept throughout their lifetime for survival.

To prevent the diabetic complication, patients with type 1 diabetes require a strict control of blood glucose level.

Although type 1 diabetes can be diagnosed at any age, it is one of the most common chronic diseases of childhood. Its prevalence increases between the ages 5 and 7 years or near puberty [1].

It has been reported that the incidence of type 1 diabetes is increasing worldwide for several decades [2] and it is likely to have been most pronounced in children aged 4 years and younger [3]. If these trends continue, the total prevalence of people with type 1 diabetes will increase in the coming years [4].

A continuous hyperglycemia in type 1 diabetes leads to various chronic complications. Recently, official healthcare providers have paid more attention to the prevention of disabling chronic complications, such as diabetic retinopathy, nephropathy, neuropathy, and atherosclerosis with cardiovascular disease, and much more attention has been paid for adverse bone metabolism in type 1 diabetes. [5] In this review, we provide a brief overview on the effects of type 1 diabetes on both bone in general and hard tissue in craniofacial region.

2. General effects of type 1 diabetes on bone

The relation between diabetes and bone metabolism has been considered for a long time; however, many questions still remain hidden and unclear. Pathophysiology of diabetes arises from the insufficient insulin action, and such insulin action may have an influence on the bone metabolism directly or indirectly. Clinically, it is well known that type 1 and type 2 diabetes are involved in an increased risk of fractures [6, 7]; on the other hand, bone mineral density

(BMD) is decreased in type 1 diabetes than in type 2 diabetes [7]. The reasons for this discrepancy are not fully understood. Indeed both type 1 and type 2 diabetes are the same in terms of an abnormal glucose tolerance, but pathological condition is different. In this part, we discuss diabetic osteopenia in type 1 diabetes from the viewpoints of insulin deficiency and hyperglycemia.

2.1. Insulin deficiency and bone metabolism

It is widely recognized that bone volume and bone quality are decreased in type 1 diabetes patients, and it is thought that insulin has a pivotal role in bone formation [7]. In animal experiment, streptozotocin (STZ)-induced type 1 diabetes rat or mouse showed a decrease in bone volume (BV) and bone fragility by the decrease of bone formation [8–10].

In insulin receptor substrate-1 (IRS-1)-deficient mouse, osteoblast differentiation and function were impaired, and as a result, there is a decrease in BV [11].

Remarkable hyperglycemia exists with insulin deficiency in the type 1 diabetes model animals, and it seems to be thought that not only the insulin deficiency but also the hyperglycemic condition gives some influences on bone metabolism. On the other hand, it appears that decrease in anabolic action at the osteoblasts level in type 1 diabetes is the main cause of the bone metabolism disorder by serial animal experiments in which the disorder of glucose metabolism is slight under the normal breeding condition in IRS-1- or IRS-2-deficient mice. On the basis of these findings, one should consider the rise in onset, osteoporosis, and bone fracture frequency of the osteoporosis in type 1 diabetes mellitus depends on an osteoplasty disorder by the insulin deficiency.

2.2. Bone Mineral Density (BMD) in type 1 diabetes

In 1948, Albright and Reifenstein described for the first time the association between diabetes and reduced bone mass [12]. In 1976, Levin et al. demonstrated that almost 50% of the patients with type 1 diabetes had a reduction of BMD at the wrist [13]. Since then, many papers have been published. BMD seems to be reduced in patients with type 1 diabetes in most [14–17], but not all [18, 19]. The studies concerning the bone metabolism in type 1 diabetes can be categorized into two groups: 1) studies evaluating bone metabolism in diabetic children and adolescents who did not reach the peak of bone mass yet and 2) studies evaluating bone metabolism in adults who developed type 1 diabetes after having reached peak of bone mass.

It seems to be difficult to study bone metabolism in such population as children/adolescents whose skeleton is still in the way of growing. Moreover, the majority of studies included the children/adolescents at different stage of puberty and, therefore, at different stages of acquisition of bone mass. This probably has been one of the main reasons for the lack of concordant results about the impact of diabetes on growing bones.

Some reports showed no differences in BMD between type 1 diabetic children/adolescents and their peer without diabetes [20–26]. However, in other studies, low bone mineral content (BMC) and low BMD both at spine and at femoral neck in type 1 diabetic children/adolescents

[27–33] have been described. Moreover, some longitudinal studies demonstrated a significant reduction of either lumber spine or femoral neck BMD in diabetic patients after 2–4 years of follow-up, despite normal BMD at baseline [20, 23]. Therefore, it seems that type 1 diabetes, appeared in childhood, may alter the acquisition of bone mass that can be registered in youth ages or later in adult life.

Indeed, the majority of studies, performed on the type 1 diabetes adults, consistently showed a reduction of BMD either at lumbar spine and/or at femur [34, 35, 36–40]. Only a few studies [41–43], which were conducted on small groups of diabetic patients (less than 40 cases), were discordant. Vestergaard et al. [44] having analyzed 80 studies regarding bone density in diabetes has proved in his meta-analysis that type 1 diabetes patients have lower BMD than the people without diabetes. Frequency of reduced BMD in type 1 diabetes varies largely from 3 to 40% [36–40]. Eller-Vainicher et al. [45] reported that about 30% of 175 type 1 diabetes patients had low bone mass (osteopenia/osteoporosis) at spine and/or femur, which was significantly higher in comparison with healthy controls.

2.3. Fracture risk in type 1 diabetes

In type 1 diabetes patients, the frequency of lifetime fractures at any site has been reported to be increased as compared to counterparts without diabetes. The meta-analysis of Vestergaard et al. [44] demonstrated a 6.94-fold increased risk of hip fracture in type 1 diabetes. Further, *Zhukouskaya et al.* [45] reported that type 1 diabetes patients were found to have an increased prevalence of asymptomatic vertebral fractures as well, which have been observed in 25% of diabetic subjects. In conclusion, there is strong evidence that bones in type 1 diabetes patients are characterized by poor mineralization and smaller and thinner size with reduced bone strength and quality, which can lead to a higher fracture incidence at any site, predominantly at femoral neck.

2.4. Association between hyperglycemia and bone metabolism in diabetes

Type 1 diabetes is caused by absolute lack of insulin, and insulin has anabolic effect on bone. However, not only insulin but also hyperglycemia has some influence on the bone metabolism. In in vivo study, it is difficult to evaluate the influence on bone metabolism by hyperglycemia or insulin deficiency separately, so the influence of hyperglycemia on bone is considered at a cell level mainly.

In an experiment of osteoblastic cell, it was reported that the differentiation and function of osteoblastic cell were suppressed under osmolality-adjusted hyperglycemic condition [46].

In our previous experiment using MC3T3-E1 cell line, osteoblastic cells were cultured in medium containing normal (5.6 mM) or high (10, 20, or 30 mM) glucose with or without bone morphogenic protein 2 (BMP-2). Runx2 mRNA expression, which is a key transcription factor associated with osteoblast differentiation, was affected by glucose concentration and culture duration independently of the absence or presence of BMP-2 in the culture. (Fig. 1) [47]. Moreover, we could find both GLP-1 receptor (GLP-1R) and GIP receptor (GIPR) m RNA expression in osteoblastic cell first time ever (Fig. 2), and mRNA expression level of GLP-1R and GIPR were regulated by glucose concentrations in cells undergoing the differentiation induced by BMP-2 (Figs. 3, 4). GLP-1 or GIP belong to the incretin family. They both play important roles in regulating insulin secretion from pancreatic β-cells. GIPR and GLP-1R, the receptors of GIP and GLP-1, are expressed in various tissues, with a significant amount expressed in pancreas. Previous reports showed that GIPR is expressed in osteoblastic cells, but no study regarding GLP-1R expression had been conducted [48]. Although osteoblastic cells were thought to express a functional receptor for GLP-1, there is no direct evidence for the mRNA and protein expression of GLP-1R in these cells. GIP is known to have direct effects on bone, whereas the effects of GLP-1 on bone metabolism are mediated by thyroid hormone. [49] Our RT-PCR analysis revealed that MC3T3-E1 cells express GLP-1R and GIPR, suggesting that GLP-1 may directly affect bone, similar to GIP (Fig. 4). GLP-1R and GIPR are well-known G protein-coupled receptor (GPCR) and are potential targets for drug discovery [47]. It has been reported that the administration of insulin and thiazolidinediones increases fracture risk, whereas inhibitors of dipeptidyl peptidase-4 (DPP-4) were associated with reduced fracture risk. DPP-4 inactivates GLP-1, and its inhibitors improve glycemic control in patients with type 2 diabetes by preventing incretin degradation [50]. These findings show that GLP-1R links bone metabolism and glucose metabolism in osteoblasts and that GLP-1 might be a potential therapeutic target in bone diseases.

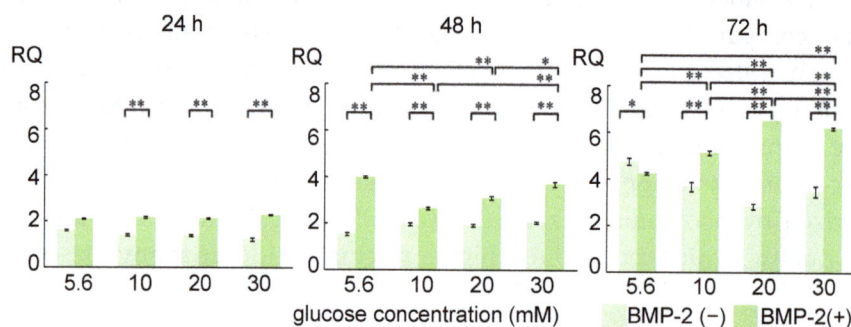

Figure 1. Effects of the glucose concentration on Runx2 mRNA expression. MC3T3-E1 cells were cultured in medium containing 5.6 (normal), or 10, 20, and 30 mM (high) concentrations of glucose in the absence or presence of bone morphogenetic protein-2 (BMP-2). Runx2 mRNA expression was determined after 24, 48, and 72 h of culture. Values are the means ± standard error of the mean (SEM) ($n = 4$/group). *$P < 0.05$ and **$P < 0.01$.

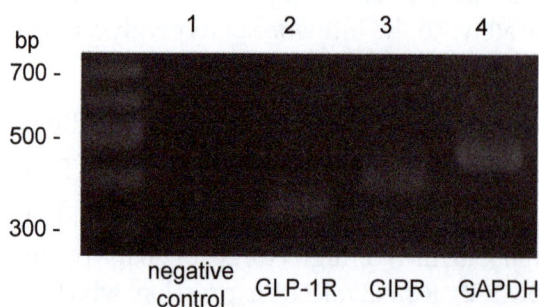

Figure 2. Reverse transcriptase-polymerase chain reaction (RT-PCR) analysis of glucagon-like peptide-1 receptor (GLP-1R) and glucose-dependent insulinotropic polypeptide receptor (GIPR) mRNA expression in MC3T3-E1 cells. Lane 1, negative control; lane 2, GLP-1R (337 bp); lane 3, GIPR (382 bp); lane 4, GAPDH (452 bp).

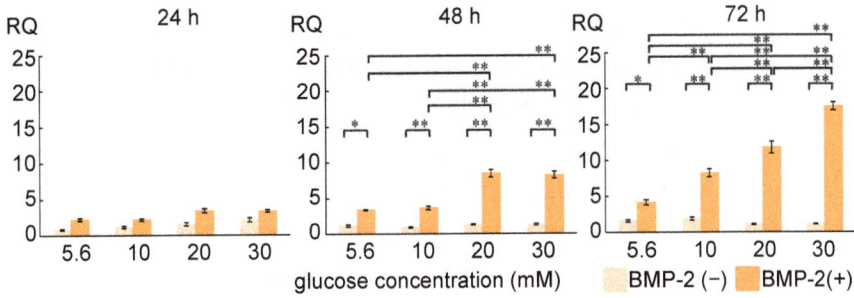

Figure 3. Effects of the glucose concentration on glucagon-like peptide-1 receptor (GLP-1R) mRNA expression. MC3T3-E1 cells were cultured in medium containing 5.6 (normal), or 10, 20 and 30 mM (high) concentrations of glucose in the absence or presence of bone morphogenetic protein-2 (BMP-2). GLP-1R mRNA expression after 24, 48, and 72 h of culture. Values are the means ± standard error of the mean (SEM) ($n = 4$/group). *$P < 0.01$.

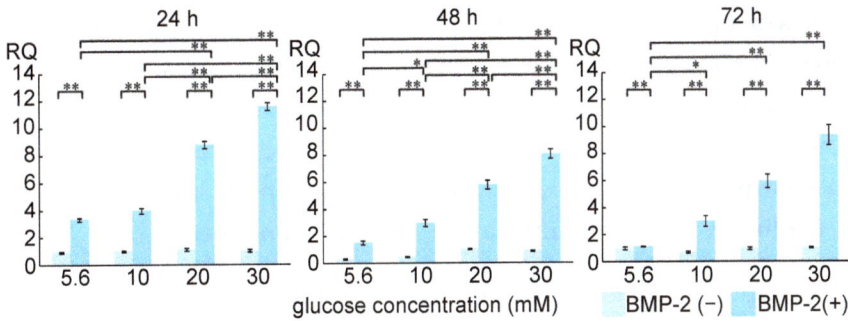

Figure 4. Effects of glucose concentration on glucose- dependent insulinotropic polypeptide receptor (GIPR) mRNA expression. MC3T3-E1 cells were cultured in medium containing 5.6 (normal), or 10, 20, and 30 mM (high) concentrations of glucose in the absence or presence of bone morphogenetic protein-2 (BMP-2). GIPR mRNA expression after 24, 48, and 72 h of culture. Values are the means ± standard error of the mean (SEM) ($n = 4$/group). *$P < 0.01$.

3. Effect of type 1 diabetes on craniofacial complex

Diabetes is one of the systemic diseases affecting a considerable number of patients worldwide [51]. Numerous clinical and experimental studies on the complications of diabetes have demonstrated extensive alterations in bone and mineral metabolism, linear growth, and body composition [52]. As we mentioned in the previous section, depletion of insulin in type 1 diabetes causes a reduction of bone composition, delay in fracture healing, and reduction of BMD in general. A long list of literature was dedicated to study the influence or complications of type 1 diabetes on general bones. However, there are few reports discussing the effects of type 1 diabetes on the craniofacial complex which is regulated by hormones, nutrients, mechanical forces, and various peripheral growth factors.

In craniofacial region, it is well known that bone metabolism in growth period is really intricate because there are mosaic growth sites where bones grow at different rates or mature at different times, which also depend on each individual's growth stage, and the response to growth disruption is much more complicated than that of the appendicular skeleton. There are a few studies diabetes may significantly affect the bone remodeling process which is observed during treatments involving the application of mechanical or functional force to the craniofacial complex and the teeth as those applied during orthodontic tooth movement. Moreover, it is likely that the type 1 diabetes may have altered the growth of patients due to insulin deficiency and consequently led to skeletal mutation is it mutation or maturation?

Type 1 diabetes is well recognized in the endocrine disorders,, and a peak of onset is concentrated in childhood and adolescence, characterized by hyperglycemia as a cardinal biochemical feature that leads to several impairment of physical and emotional developments. There are some reports focusing on the altered bone remodeling in type 1 diabetes, which indicates the reduction of osteoblast activity or function. Bone mass decrease and rate of bone fracture risk increase have been often seen in type 1 diabetes patients. Impaired glucose metabolism results in adverse effects on bone metabolism, especially in type 1 diabetes patients who suffer from decreased bone mineral density (BMD) and increased risk of fractures. The pathophysiological mechanisms of increased risk of fracture in diabetes patients are divided into two reasons: osteopenia caused by decreased BMD and increased risk of fall and traumas caused by peripheral diabetic neuropathy. However, there are few reports about hard tissue in craniofacial region, in other words, cranium, maxilla, mandible, and teeth.

The aim of this chapter is to discuss the complexity of the dento-alveolar system and how it was affected by type 1 diabetes.

3.1. Effect of type 1 diabetes on bone in craniofacial region

There are two processes of bone formation: "intramembranous ossification" and "endochondral ossification." Endochondral ossification is a cartilage bone formation and it occurs in a replacement process within the cartilage models of the embryo and infant. Intramembranous bone forms through the activation of the osteoblastic cell or specialized bone forming cell in one of the layers of the fetal-connective tissue. The bones of the cranial vault, the face, and the clavicle are formed by the style of intramembranous ossification. All the other bones are formed in the manner of cartilage ossification. The bones formed by intramembranous ossification are the mandible, the maxilla, the premaxilla, the frontal bone, the palatine bone, the squamous part of temporal bone, the zygomatic bone, the medial plate of the pterygoid process, the vomer, the tympanic part of the temporal bone, the nasal bone, the lacrimal bone, and the parietal bone. The original pattern of intramembranous bone changes with progressive maturative growth when these bones begin to adapt to environmental influences. This accounts for deformities due to malfunction, disease, and other environmental factor [53].

3.2. Causes of general growth problems

It is thought that growth disturbance can be associated with specific anatomic or functional defects. Some kinds of endocrinal or metabolic disorders are known to cause a systemic growth disorder. Also, genetic, nutritional, or environmental factor can be the causes of growth disturbance. Disturbances in somatic growth show themselves in retardation or acceleration of the skeletal system, including the facial and cranial bones. Causes of growth problems usually fall into the following categories [54]:

• familial short stature;

• constitutional growth delay with delayed adolescence or delayed maturation;

• illness that affects the whole body (systemic disease);

• endocrine disease (hormonal disorder); and

• congenital problems in the tissues where growth occurs.

3.3. Effect of type 1 diabetes on bone and growth

Concerning juvenile diabetes, previous report about hand-wrist radiographs [55]. showed that usually, there is a delay in the development of appearance or ossification center of the carpal bone. These defects seem to occur twice as frequently in boys than in girls, and the total incidence of juvenile diabetes patients with abnormalities and developmental disorders was 24.3%. There was also a delay in the growth of bone, in 51% of diabetic males and in 60% of diabetic females. The trend of growth retardation in bone was large. The longer the disease duration of diabetes, the shorter the bone growth will be. Bone mass reduction in diabetic patients has been explained by the decrease in the proliferative capacity of fibroblasts. In addition, premature aging of all cells has been suggested as the basis for diabetes problems, which is believed to lead to early osteopenia. The yearly bone loss was reported to be 1.35% in patients with type 1 diabetes [56]. Moreover, reduction rate of bone mineral, along with the condition worsened in diabetes, was significantly faster despite of an increase in insulin dosage, when compared with patients with unchanged or improved insulin secretion. It was considered that exogenous insulin administration cannot fully compensate for the decrease in the endogenous insulin secretion. In addition, according to these studies, the bone resorption in patients with type 1 diabetes were increased, and vitamin D_3 deficiency associated with the disease were not observed. Vertebral bone density has been studied in type 1 diabetic children [56]. In diabetic children, it has been found that the cortical bone density decreases slightly but significantly compared with control. The decrease in the cortical bone mineral density in diabetes did not correlate with age, gender, the duration of the diabetes, or glycosylated hemoglobin concentration. These results suggested that in children with uncomplicated type 1 diabetes, decreased vertebral bone density is a minor abnormality that affects only cortical bone [55].

3.4. Outline of studying the effect of type 1 diabetes on craniofacial growth

To examine the dynamic bone metabolism and structure of craniofacial bone in diabetes, it is critically important in understanding the growth aspect and bone metabolism of the mandible. The next parts of this chapter are trying to focus on the following points:

1. The effects of juvenile diabetes on general craniofacial growth and skeletal maturation.

2. Analysis of the pattern of association between craniofacial morphology and skeletal maturation.

3. Determination of the mineral apposition rate and the bone formation rate in diabetic rat mandible using histomorphometric analysis.

4. Analysis of the diabetic effects on tooth (enamel and dentin formation).

3.5. Experimental rat model for type 1 diabetes

It is well known that the streptozotocin-induced diabetic rat and the spontaneously diabetic BioBreeding rat were used as experimental type 1 diabetic models [57]. Pathogenesis of altered bone formation in long bones after inducing type 1 diabetes with streptozotocin (STZ) has been well documented [58, 59]. Streptozotocin-induced diabetes mellitus (STZ-DM) caused by the destruction of pancreatic β-cells and is similar to type 1 diabetes in human. It is characterized by mild-to-moderate hyperglycemia, glucosuria, polyphagia, hypoinsulinemia, hyperlipidemia, and weight loss. STZ-DM also exhibits many of the complications observed in human DM including enhanced susceptibility to infection and cardiovascular disease, retinopathy, alterations in angiogenesis, delayed wound healing, diminished growth factor expression, and reduced bone formation. [60].

3.6. Induction of type 1 diabetic condition in animal experiment

We studied various changes on craniofacial hard tissue under DM condition using streptozotocin (STZ)-induced DM rat model. Three-week-old male Wistar rats (n = 12) were used for this study. They were randomly divided into two groups, the control group and the diabetes group (DM group), and each group consists of six rats. The rats in the control group were injected intraperitoneally with a single dose of 0.1M sodium citrate buffer (pH 4.5), while the rats in the DM group were injected intraperitoneally with a single dose of citrate buffer containing 60 mg/kg body weight of STZ (Sigma Chemical Co., St. Louis, MO, USA) [58, 61–63]. All animals were fed on standard rodent diet (Rodent Diet CE-2; Japan Clea Inc., Shizuoka, Japan) with free access to water. Body weights, the presence of glucose in urine, and blood glucose levels were recorded on days 0, 2, 7, 14, 21, and 28 after STZ injection. Diabetes condition was determined by the presence of glucose in urine and blood. The urine of the rats was tested using reagent strips (Uriace Ga; TERUMO) [64, 65]. Blood samples of the rats were obtained via vein puncture of a tail vein, and blood glucose levels were determined using a glucometer (Ascensia Brio; Bayer Medical). Rats with a positive urine test and a blood glucose level greater than 200 mg/dl were considered as diabetic. Time course of the animal experiment is shown in Fig. 5.

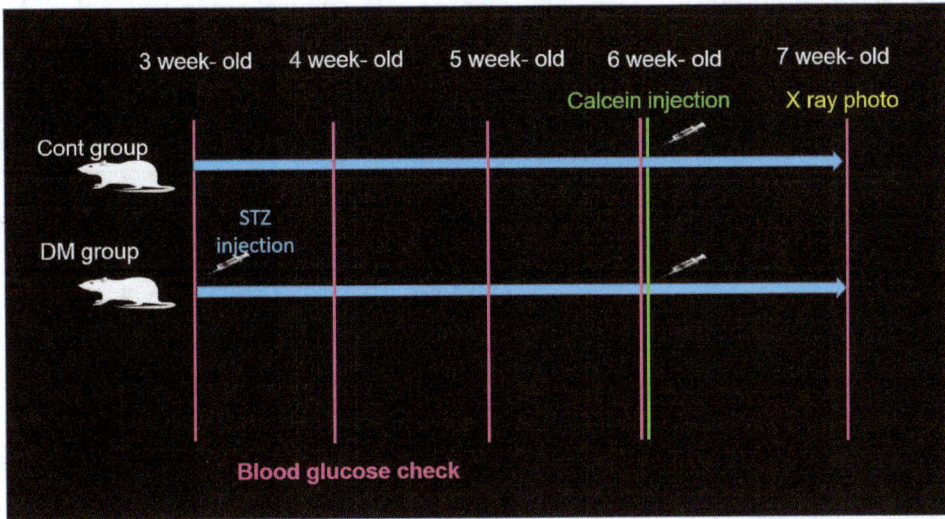

Figure 5. The time schedule of experiment

3.7. Evaluating the effect of type 1 diabetes on craniofacial growth in rat

Cephalometric analysis

Cephalometric measurements are still one of the most widely spread diagnostic aids crucial for the diagnosis of various abnormalities in the craniofacial complex [66].

The protocol for examining the cephalometric measurements in Type 1 diabetic rats involved the following steps:

1. Prior to each radiographic session, the rats were anesthetized with diethyl ether and intraperitoneally injected with 8% chloral hydrate using 0.5 ml/100 g of body weight.

2. After anesthesia, the rats were placed in the same way using specially designed apparatus to maintain standardized head posture and contact with the film (SGP-3; Mitsutoyo, Tokyo, Japan) where the head of each rat was fixed firmly with a pair of ear rods oriented vertically to the sagittal plane, and the incisors were fixed into a plastic ring. The settings of lateral and dorsoventral cephalometric radiographs were 50/55 kVp, 15/10 mA, and 20/60-sec impulses, respectively [68].

3. Then, a 10-mm steel calibration rod was incorporated into the clear acrylic table on which the animals were positioned for the radiographs.

All the radiographs were developed and scanned at high resolution by the same operator (Fig. 6). The cephalometric landmarks were derived from previous studies on rodents [68–70]. The selected linear measurements were then obtained (Table 1). To ensure reliability and reproducibility of each measurement, each distance was digitized twice and the two values were averaged. In our studies, evaluation of the craniofacial growth of diabetic rats at the age of 7 weeks was carried out using lateral and dorsoventral cephalometric radiographs. All of the data in each experiment were confirmed for the normal distribution; that is, Student's t-test was used to compare the mean of each data recorded in the control group and in the DM group. All statistical analyses were performed at a 5% significance level using statistic software (v. 10; SPSS, Chicago, IL, USA).

Neurocranium	Mandible
Po–N: total skull length	Go–Mn: posterior corpus length
Po–E: cranial vault length	Ml–Il: anterior corpus length
Ba–E: total cranial base length	Co–Il: total mandibular length
So–E: anterior cranial base length	Co–Gn: ramus height
Ba–CB1: occipital bone length	**Transverse X-ray**
CB1'–CB2: sphenoid bone length	Go1–Go2: bigonial width
Ba–So: posterior cranial base length	C1–C2: maximum cranial width
Po–Ba: posterior neurocranium height	P1–P2: palatal width
Viscerocranium	Z1–Z2: bizygomatic width
E–N: nasal length	
Mu2–Iu: palate length	
CB2–Iu: midface length	
E–Mu1: viscerocranial height	

Table 1. Measurements of craniofacial skeleton

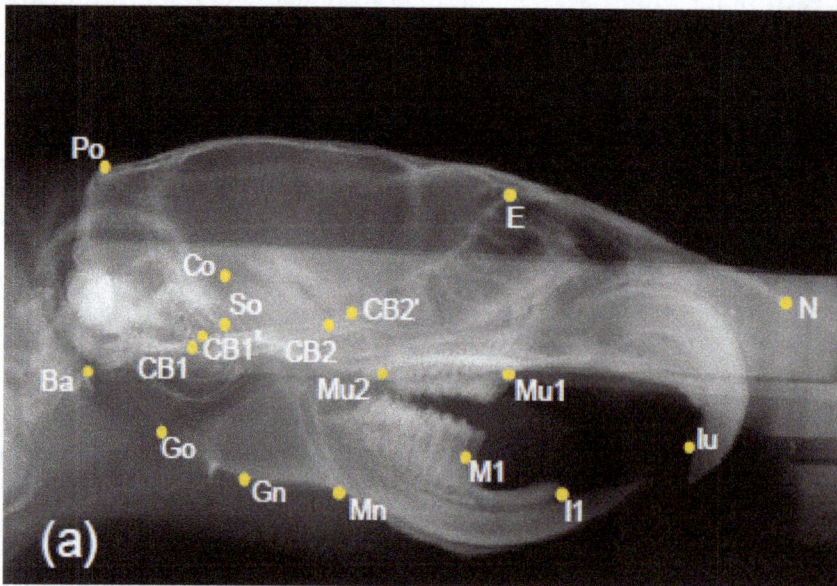

Figure 6. Location of lateral cephalometric points on radiographs: (a) sagittal

3.7.1. Changes in the total skull

The size of total skull, denoted by Po-N, was found to be significantly smaller in the DM group than in the control group (Fig. 7).

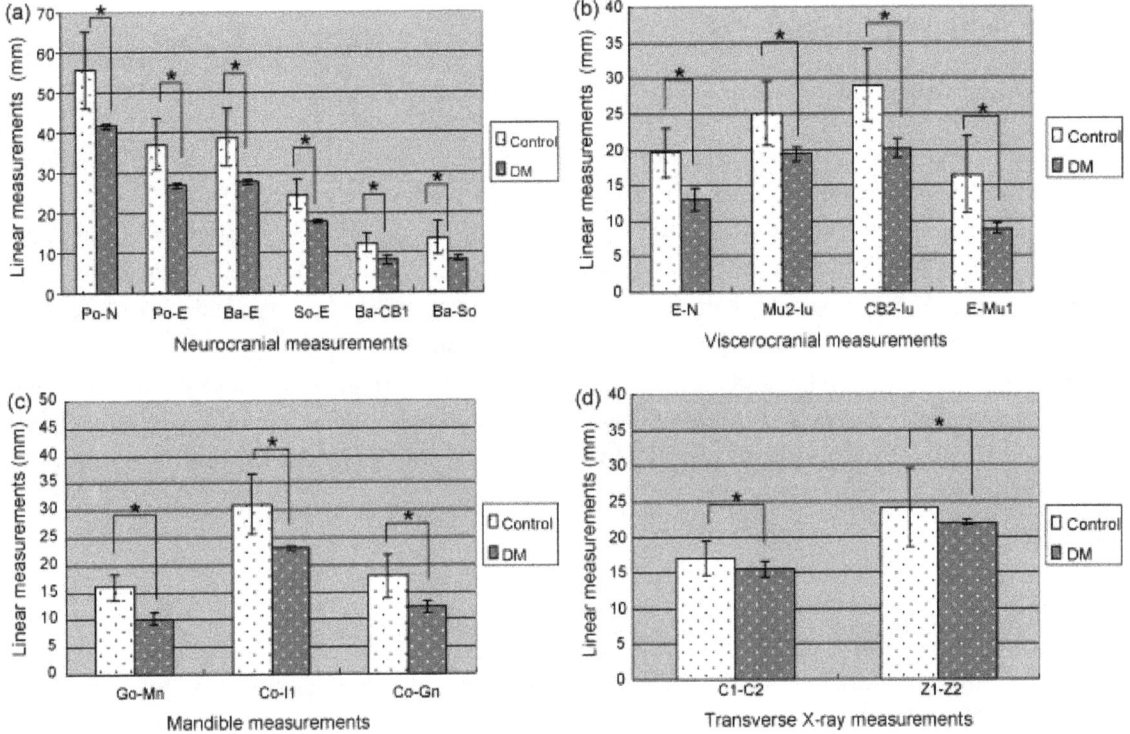

Figure 7. (A) Changes in the neurocranial measurements of the control and type 1 diabetes (DM) group. All the significant measurements are shown in this figure. Values are mean ± S.D. Significant differences between the two groups are marked with asterisks (*P* < 0.05). (B) Changes in the viscerocranial measurements of the control and DM groups. All the viscerocranial measurements are significant. Values are mean ± S.D. Significant differences between the two groups are marked with asterisks (*P* < 0.05). (C) Changes in the mandible measurements of the control and DM groups. Values are mean ± S.D. Significant differences between the two groups are marked with asterisks (*P* < 0.05). (D) Changes in the transverse X-ray measurements of the control and DM groups. Two measurements in the transverse X-ray were significant. Values are mean ± S.D. Significant differences between the two groups are marked with asterisks (*P* < 0.05).

3.7.2. Changes observed in the Neurocranium

Cranial vault length (Po-E), total cranial base length (Ba-E), anterior cranial base length (SoE), occipital bone length (Ba-CB1), and posterior cranial base length (Ba-So) were significantly shorter in DM group (Fig. 7), while the other dimensions showed no significant differences.

3.7.3. Changes in the Viscerocranium

All measurements of the viscerocranium, including the nasal length (E-N), palatal length (Mu2-Iu), midface length (CB2-Iu), and viscerocranial height (E-Mu1), showed a statistically significant decrease in DM group (Fig. 7).

3.7.4. Changes in the Mandible

In the DM group, the posterior corpus length (Go-Mn), total mandibular length (Co-Il), and the ramus height (Co-Gn) were significantly shorter than in the control group (Fig. 7); on the other hand, there were no statistical differences in the remaining dimensions.

3.8. Histomorphometric analysis of mandible

3.8.1. Fluorescent dyes used for double labeling in histomorphometric analysis

Fluorochromes are calcium-binding substances that are preferentially taken up at the site of active mineralization of bone known as the calcification front, thus labeling sites of new bone formation. They are detected using fluorescent microscopy on undecalcified sections. Labeling bones with fluorochrome markers provides a means to study the dynamics of bone formation. The rate and extent of bone deposition and resorption can be determined using double- and triple-fluorochrome labeling sequences. The sequential use of fluorochromes of clearly contrasting colors permits a more detailed record of events relating to calcification. Fluorochromes commonly used in mammals include tetracycline, calcein green, xylenol orange, alizarin red, and hematoporphyrin. Calcein gives bright green fluorescence when combined with calcium [71].

3.8.2. Calcein administrations and sections preparation

The detection of the double labeling involves the following steps:

- Rats are subcutaneously injected with 50 mg/kg body weight calcein fluorescent marker on day 21 and day 28 after STZ injection [72]. The time difference between the two injections was one week to be able to compare the amount of bone formed during this period (Fig. 8).

- All animals were sacrificed by transcardiac perfusion under deep anesthesia using 4% paraformaldehyde in 0.1 M phosphate buffer (pH 7.4).

- Mandibles were dissected and fixed in the same solution for 24 h and embedded in polystyrene resin (Rigolac; Nisshin EM Co. Ltd., Tokyo, Japan).

- Undermineralized ground frontal sections were processed to show the crown and both apices of buccal and lingual roots of the lower second molar [72].

3.8.3. Method of analysis of "Mineral Appositional Rate" and "Bone Formation Rate"

The bone around the lower second molar is centrally located within the mandibular arch, and the parallel alignment of the buccal and lingual roots is used as a precise reference when frontal sections are produced [73]. To conduct the histomorphometric analysis, it is essential to use a digitizing morphometry system to measure bone formation indices. The system consists of a confocal laser scanning microscope (LSM510; Carl Zeiss Co. Ltd., Jena, Germany) and a morphometry program (LSM Image Browser; Carl Zeiss Co. Ltd., Jena, Germany). Bone formation indices of the periosteal surfaces of the alveolar/jaw bone include mineral apposition

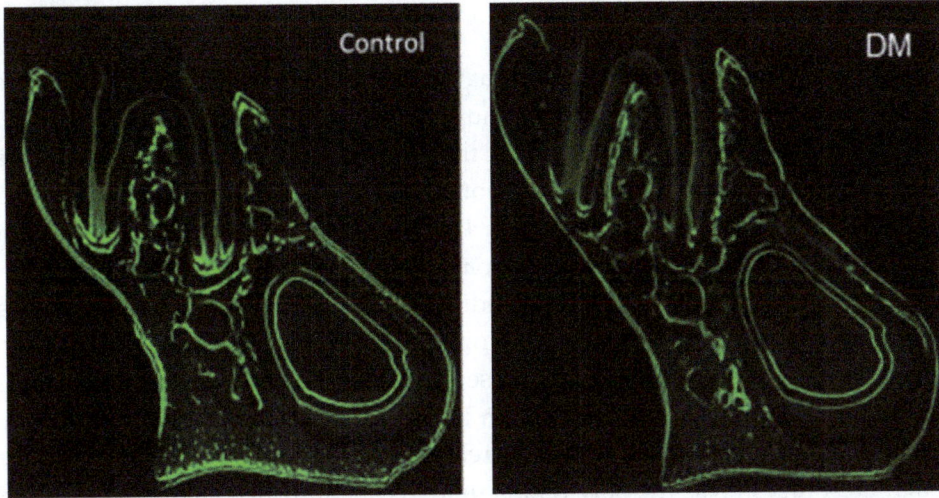

Figure 8. Frontal sections of the rat's mandibular second molar area. Control, control rat; DM, type 1 diabetes rat. Fluorescent labeling on the periosteal surface indicates new bone formation.

rate (μm/day) and bone formation rate (μm^3/μm^2/day), according to the standard nomenclature described by Parfitt and colleagues [74]. The calcein-labeled surface (CLS, in mm) is calculated as the sum of the length of double labels plus one half of the length of single labels (sL) along the entire endosteal or periosteal bone surfaces; that is, CLS = dL + 0.5sL [75]. The mineral apposition rate (MAR, in μm/day) is determined by dividing the mean of the width of the double labels by the interlabel time (7 days). The bone formation rate (BFR) is calculated by multiplying MAR by CLS [76]. Based on the reference line along the long axis of the buccal root, the area superior to the root apex was considered as an alveolar bone, while the area inferior to the root apex was considered as the jaw bone. The lingual side of the bone was excluded, because the existence of the incisor root might influence bone formation. The periosteal surfaces of the mandible were divided into four regions for analysis (Fig. 9).

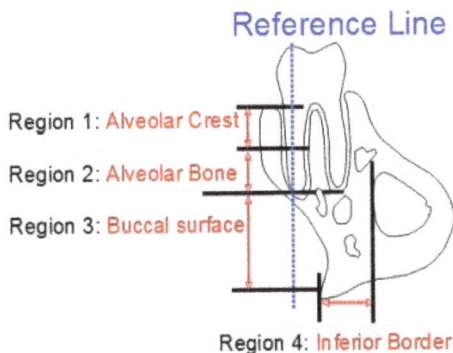

Figure 9. Schematic drawing of observation regions for dynamic bone histomorphometry. The periosteal surfaces were delimited into four areas: alveolar crest (region 1), alveolar bone (region 2), buccal surface of the jaw bone (region 3), and inferior border of the jaw bone (region 4).

3.8.4. Hitromorphometric indices

The obtained results in our study showed that in the alveolar bone (region 2), there was a significant decrease in the MAR (Fig. 10A) and the BFR (Fig. 10B) recorded in the DM group compared to the control group. However, in the alveolar crest (region 1), the MAR and the BFR in the control and the DM groups were not significantly different ($P < 0.05$). In the buccal surface (region 3) and inferior borders (region 4) of the jaw bone, the MAR (Fig. 10A) and BFR (Fig. 10B) were significantly suppressed compared with those in the control group ($P < 0.05$). Most of the periosteal surfaces in the mandibular regions of the control group showed significantly higher values recorded for the mineral apposition rate and the bone formation rate when compared to the DM group. These results agree with the previous studies that recorded diminished lamellar bone formation in DM rats' femur and may suggest an association between the DM condition and the decreased number and function of osteoblasts [61]. The alveolar crest region was the only region that did not show a significant difference in the MAR and the BFR parameters between the two groups; this may be attributed to the unique nature of this region exhibiting a highly intensive bone remodeling process especially during the teeth eruption that decreases toward the base of the socket [77]; however, further studies are needed to elaborate the detailed pattern of bone growth at the alveolar crest region.

3.9. Evaluating the type 1 diabetic effects on tooth

Type 1 diabetes exhibits various detrimental alterations on bones, and mineral metabolism [52, 58, 75]. However, there is scant information available on the possible effects exerted by the diabetic condition on tooth development and mineral content. Various clinical studies reported high caries prevalence in diabetic children when compared with healthy controls [78]. Previous studies suggested that the aforementioned increase in caries prevalence associated with type 1 diabetes may be due to alteration in the salivary gland functions resulting in decreased salivary flow. Alternative speculations were that type 1 diabetes produced increased salivary glucose levels which may have increased permeability of the parotid gland basement membrane to the elevated blood glucose. Understanding the factors contributing to the increased caries susceptibility of young patients suffering from the diabetic condition, especially young orthodontic patients who have high probability for the development of caries during their orthodontic treatment, may help dentists to plan suitable strategies for protecting such patients against the expected caries challenges. Moreover, it is of prime importance for dentists and orthodontists to explore any factors that might affect the dental tissues growth and thus the size of the teeth, which has a strong impact on the orthodontic treatment planning. Our study has employed the non-destructive micro-computed tomography (micro-CT) to examine the influence of induced type 1 diabetes on enamel and dentine mineral density and thickness using an experimental rat model. Micro-CT uses a focused beam to provide higher resolution on small samples in vitro. This method has been frequently used in experiments exploring bone and is considered as a promising technique for the assessment of tooth mineral density. In addition, a histomorphometric study was conducted to determine the effect of the type 1 diabetes condition on dentine formation and dentine mineral apposition rates in the continuously growing lower incisors of Wistar rats. This is an appropriate model for examining the

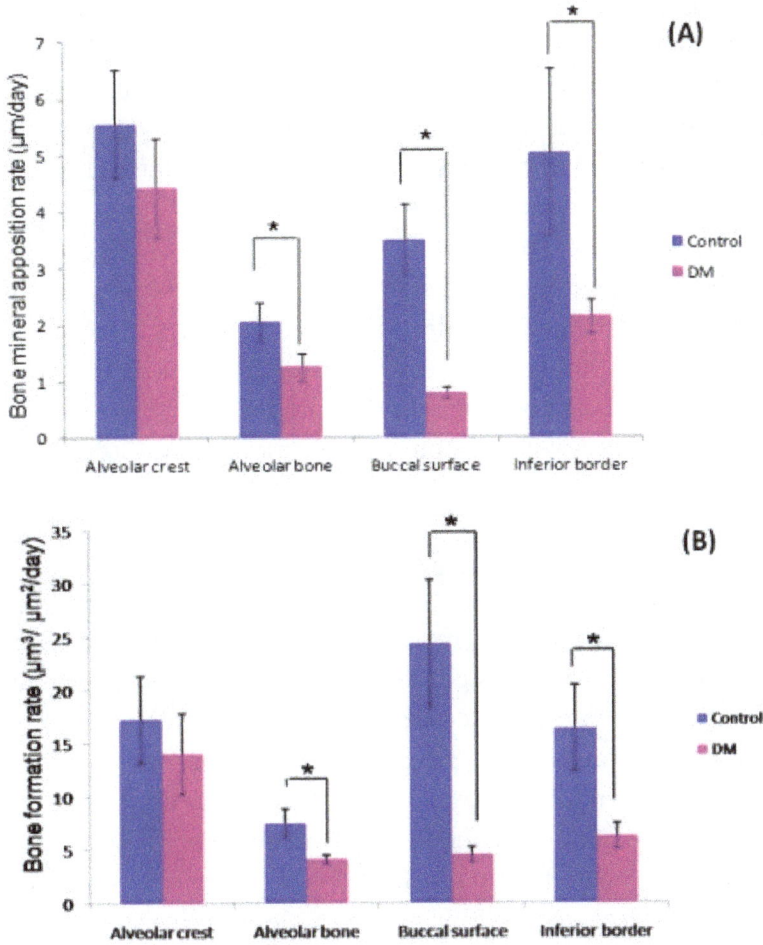

Figure 10. (A) Changes in the mineral apposition rate (MAR) of the mandible between the control group (red columns) and the type 1 diabetes mellitus (DM) group (blue columns). Alveolar crest (region 1, upper half of the tooth root, near the tooth crown). Alveolar bone (region 2, lower half of the tooth root, near the root apex). Buccal surface of the jaw bone (region 3). Inferior border of the jaw bone (region 4). The data are expressed as means ± S.D.; $n = 5$ for each group. Significantly different from controls, with *$P < 0.05$. (B) Changes in the bone formation rate (BFR/BS) of the mandible between the control group and the DM group. Alveolar crest (region 1, upper half of the tooth root, near the tooth crown). Alveolar bone (region 2, lower half of the tooth root, near the root apex). Buccal surface of the jaw bone (region 3). Inferior border of the jaw bone (region 4). The data are expressed as means ± S.D.; $n = 5$ for each group. Significantly different from controls, with *$P < 0.05$. In the buccal surface (region 3) and inferior borders (region 4) of the jaw bone, the MAR (Fig. 4A) and the BFR (Fig. 4B) are significantly suppressed compared with those in the control group ($P < 0.05$).

effects of different factors on the development of hard tissues. The tested null hypotheses in this study were that the type 1 diabetes condition will not adversely affect thickness, mineral density, and the rate of tissue formation and mineral apposition in enamel and dentine.

3.9.1. Calcein administration and section preparation for tooth observation

Rats were subcutaneously injected with calcein fluorescent marker (50 mg/kg body weight) on day 21 and day 28 after STZ injection. All animals were anesthetized and sacrificed by transcardiac perfusion by 4% paraformaldehyde in 0.1 M phosphate buffer (pH 7.4). The right mandibles were removed and fixed in the same solution. After being embedded in polystyrene resin (Rigolac; Nisshin EM Co. Ltd., Tokyo, Japan), undemineralized ground mesial sections were cut using water-cooled diamond saw microtome (1600 Microtome; Leitz Wetzlar, Germany) parallel to the long axis of the rat molars just 2 mm to the mesial surface of the first lower molar crown; the distal second cut was done 2 mm distal to the crown of the first molar. The specimen mesial surface was then ground flat with water-cooled silicon carbide discs (600- and 1200-grade papers; Buehler) until it was possible to observe the two mesial canals and two mesial pulp chamber horns of the first molar. The ground mesial surface was glued on a glass slide, and the same grinding procedures were repeated from the distal surface until we can observe the two mesial canals and two mesial pulp horns of the first molar from the distal side. The obtained specimen is then wet-polished using diamond paste (1 mm; Buehler) to obtain a highly polished surface.

3.9.2. Analysis of histomorphometric indices of tooth

Dentine formation indices in control and type 1 diabetes groups were determined in the crown analogue area parallel to the long axis of the mesial surface of the first molar. A digitizing morphometry system was used to measure the dentine formation indices. The system consisted of a confocal laser scanning microscope (LSM510; Carl Zeiss Co. Ltd., Jena, Germany) and a morphometry program (LSM Image Browser; Carl Zeiss Co. Ltd., Germany). Dentine formation indices included dentine mineral apposition rate (mm/day) and dentine formation rate ($\mu m^3/\mu m^2$/day). The method for the calculation of bone indices was modified from a method described by Parfitt et al. [74] The calcein-labeled dentine surface (CLS, in mm) was calculated as the sum of the length of double labels (dL) plus one half of the length of single labels (sL) along the entire dentine surface; that is, CLS = dL + 0.5sL [17]. The mineral apposition rate (MAR, in μm/day and in μm^2/day) was determined by dividing the mean of the width of the double labels by the interlabel time (7 days). The dentine formation rate (DFR) was calculated by multiplying MAR by CLS [18]. For the measurements of mineral apposition rate, the average of 3 inter-label widths at a 100-μm interval was calculated for each sample.

Green fluorescent lines labeled with calcein fluorescent marker at two different time points showed that dentine formation took place between day 21 and day 28 in the control and type 1 diabetes groups (Fig. 11A and B). In the type 1 diabetes group, there were significant decreases in both mineral apposition and dentine formation rates (Fig. 11C and D) when compared to control group ($P < 0.05$).

Furthermore, our micro-CT results (details of method not shown) revealed that there was no significant difference in the enamel and dentine mineral densities between the control and experimental diabetes groups (Fig. 12). However, the type 1 diabetes group showed a significant decrease in the thickness of enamel and dentine surfaces when compared to the control group (Fig. 13) [79].

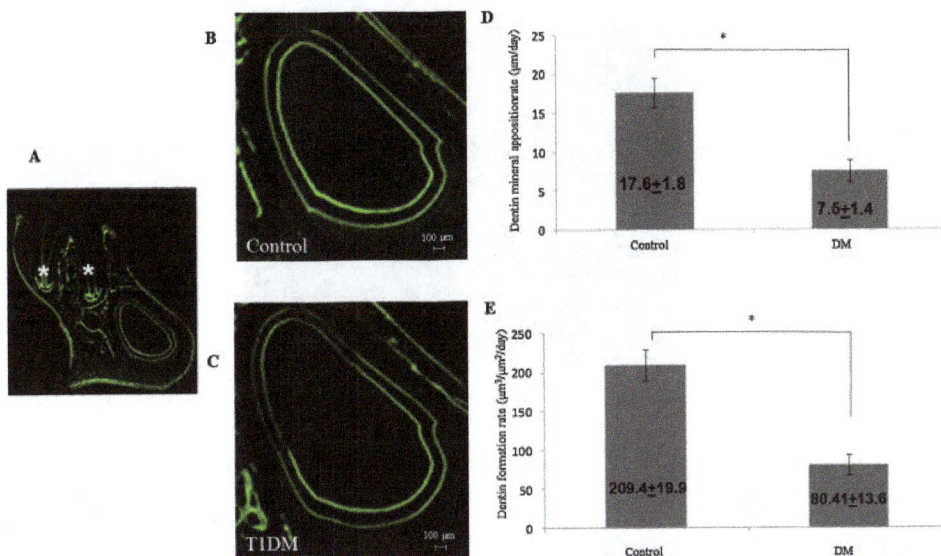

Figure 11. (A) Frontal section of the lower right mandible. *The lower first molar two roots that were considered the landmark for cutting all samples. (B, C) Frontal sections of the rat incisor mandibular first molar area. (B) Control; (C) T1DM. Fluorescent labelling indicates the new dentine formation. (D) The mineral apposition rate (MAR) of the dentine mandibular incisor for the control group and the T1DM group. The data are expressed as means ± SD. $n = 10$ for each group. Significant difference from controls, with *$P < 0.05$. (E) The dentine formation rate (DFR) of the dentine mandibular incisor for the control group and the DM group. The data are expressed as means ± S.D. $n = 10$ for each group. Significant difference from controls, with *$P < 0.05$).

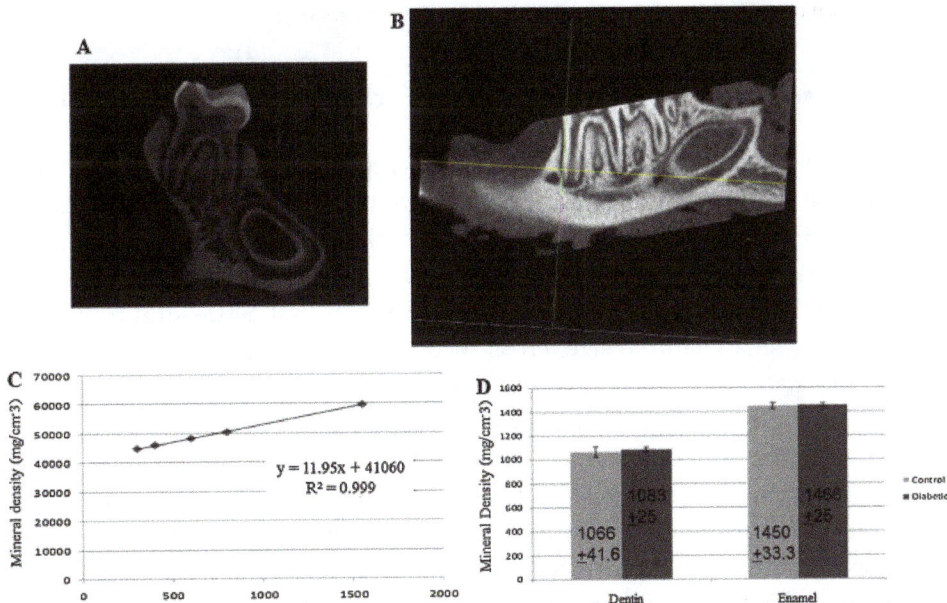

Figure 12. (A) Representative 3D reconstruction of the left mandible imaged by micro-CT. (B) The left mandible with the vertical reference line extending parallel to the mesial surface of the first molar. (C) Mineral density calibration curve based on the gray scale values obtained from the mineral reference phantoms (linear regression, R2 > 0.99). (D) Graph showing that there is no significant difference in the incisor enamel and dentine mineral densities between the control and T1DM groups.

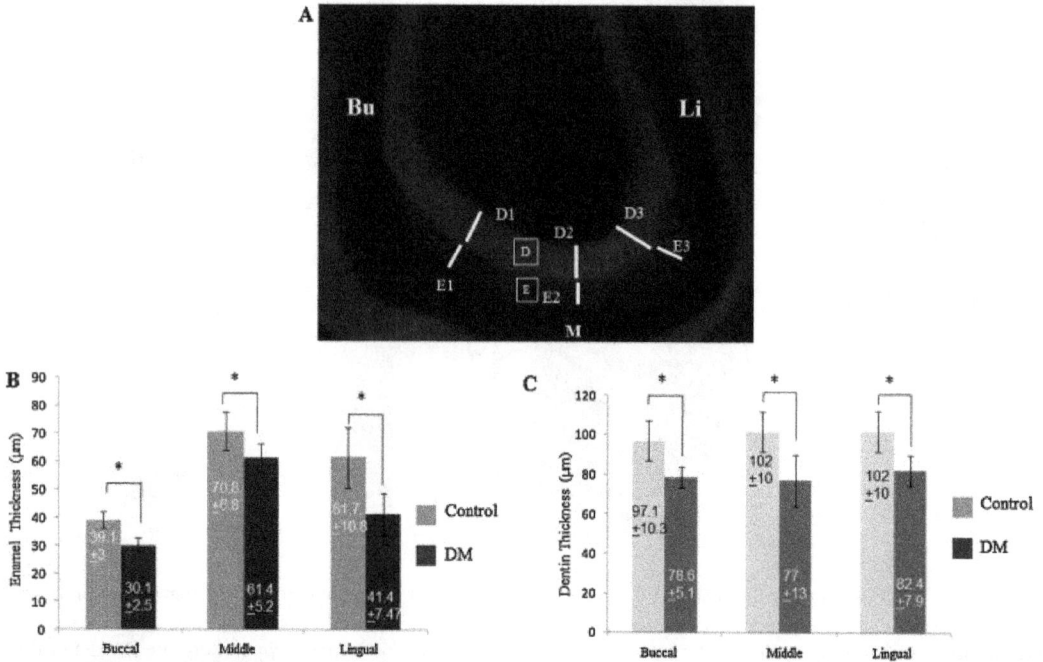

Figure 13. (A) The micro-CT oriented image of the rat mandibular incisor showing the three zones (E1–E3) selected for evaluation of enamel thickness and the three zones (D1–D3) selected for evaluation of dentine thickness. B-buccal; M-middle; Li-lingual. (B) The T1DM group shows a significant decrease in the thickness of enamel surface when compared to control group in the three different zones. (C) The T1DM group shows a significant decrease in the thickness of dentine surface when compared to control group in the three different zones ($P < 0.05$).

3.10. Suggested mechanism for the effect of diabetic condition on craniofacial complex

Growth of the craniofacial or maxillofacial complex is regulated by genetic and environmental factors [57]. For normal growth and morphogenesis of the cranial and maxillofacial complex, a proper regulation by hormones, nutrients, mechanical forces, and various general and local growth factor is essential. Type 1 diabetes causes a deteriorating growth and metabolic disorder of bone in both humans and experimental animals [58]. Since studies in humans are generally limited by small sample size, cross-sectional designs, uncontrolled variables, and often retrospective natures; it often performed more rigorous analyses using animal models [56]. We have observed the growth of the rat from 3 weeks of age to 7 weeks of age in our study. According to the previous craniofacial growth studies, this period corresponds to the initial stage of growth in humans [80, 81]. Consequently, STZ-induced DM models in our study were used to investigate the effects of type 1 diabetes on the development of craniofacial complex. These STZ-induced DM rats showed a significant reduction in the growth of a large portion of the unit of craniofacial hard tissues compared with control rats, but regarding the rest of the craniofacial skeletal units (sphenoid bone length, posterior neurocranium height, anterior corpus length, bigonial width, and palatal width), no significant difference were observed between the control and the STZ-induced DM groups. In general, craniofacial skeletal growth was significantly lower in STZ-induced DM group compared to controls in all three dimensions. The previous study investigated the DM effect exclusively on the growth of the mandible and suggested that the diabetic condition had a differential effect on the osseous components and/or its associated non-skeletal tissues. They discussed that disharmony of the mandibular growth was due to the condition of the DM, such as renal failure, anemia, body weight change, or alteration in the food-intake qualities [58]. Thus, we hypothesize that the deficiency in the craniofacial growth in our experiment might be due to the diabetic condition in the DM group as it has been reported that specific changes in bone metabolism are associated with DM. In addition, some of the pathogenic potential, insulinopenia, microvascular bone, dysregulation of mineral metabolism, changes in local factors that regulate bone remodeling, and even an intrinsic disorder related to type 1 diabetes, have been proposed [82, 83]. It is thought that the aforementioned deficiency of the insulin associated with type 1 diabetes may have a direct effect on bone metabolism. It was reported that normal insulin levels exert a direct anabolic effect on bone cells [82]. Multiple osteoblast-like cell lines, expressing the insulin receptor on the cell surface, have a high capacity for insulin binding [84]. Moreover, osteoclast are known to reduce bone resorption in response to insulin stimulation [85]. These findings support the view that insulin in bone can act directly against osteoblasts in combination with the inhibition of osteoclasts [60, 85], and this mechanism of action can be used to explain the delay in the craniofacial growth in STZ-DM. Diabetes has a detrimental effect on osseous turnover due to decreased both osteoblast and osteoclast activities and numbers and, a lower percentage of osteoid surface and osteocalcin synthesis, as well as increased time for mineralization of osteoid [82]. In a separate stage in matrix-induced endochondral bone formation, the influence of diabetes was reported to have a significant impact on the biomechanical behavior of bone. In addition, chondrogenesis and calcification of bone were reduced by 50% in diabetic animals [86]. This was also consistent with our findings that showed a significant reduction in the craniofacial linear measurements of the DM group. In addition, insulin can exert synergistic effects with other anabolic agents on bone, such as parathyroid hormone (PTH) [60, 85]. Type 1 diabetes animal models frequently show the alteration in bone turnover, retarded growth, increased concentration of PTH, and reduced concentration of 1,25-dihydroxyvitamin D [82, 87]. The effects of PTH on the bones are rather complex; PTH stimulates resorption or bone formation depending on the concentration used, the duration of the exhibition, and the administration method [82, 86, 87, 88]. Moreover, 1,25-dihydroxivitamin D, like PTH, belongs to the most important group of bone regulatory hormones. It regulates osteoclastic differentiation from hematopoietic mononuclear cells, and osteoblastic functions and activity [82, 89].

Moreover, insulin may indirectly regulate the increase in the concentration of growth hormone (GH) in serum concentration by direct regulation of the hepatic growth hormone receptor. That would result in abnormalities in the insulin growth factor-1 (IGF-1) in T1DM [90] which consequently might have led to the retarded growth in uncontrolled DM, in our study. In the present study, the mineral appositional rates and bone formation rate in DM group were significantly lower in the most area of periosteal surface in mandible as compared to the control group. These results are in agreement with the previous studies that reported diminished lamellar bone formation in DM rats' femur and may suggesting the putative association between the DM condition and the decreased number and function of osteoblasts [61]. The alveolar crest region was the only region that did not show a significant difference in the mineral apposition rate and the bone formation rate parameters between healthy and DM groups; this may be attributed to the unique nature of this region exhibiting a highly intensive bone remodeling process especially during the teeth eruption that decreases toward the base of the socket [77]. A significant decrease in bone volume fraction, trabecular thickness, and trabecular numbers was confirmed by micro-CT analysis in DM rats. DM rats also showed a significant increase in the trabecular separation and the trabecular space when compared with the control group. This finding indicated the deterioration of the bone quality in the DM group. These observations are in agreement with other works suggesting that the glycemic levels play an important role in modulating the trabecular architecture especially in mandibular bone [60]. In this context, these results may describe a state of osteopenia in experimental diabetic rats, which might be caused by an imbalance between bone formation and resorption. A histometric evaluation of bone resorption was performed by counting the number of osteoclast cells on the distal surface of the alveolar bone adjacent to the mesio-buccal root of the second molar. These evaluations revealed that the number of osteoclasts was significantly lower in the DM rats than in the controls, in line with the previous studies on DM rats' mandible and long bones [58]. These studies confirm that the decreased rate of bone turnover may be associated with the DM condition. This worsening effect of the structure and dynamic bone formation on mandible might be due to a number of pathogenic potentials such as insulinopenia, bone microangiopathy, impaired regulation of mineral metabolism, alteration in local factors that regulate bone remodeling [57, 83]. However, the adverse effects observed may not be associated with the significant loss of rats' weights observed in the diabetic group starting from day 14 because previous research [57, 60] showed that the mandibular growth was not affected in normal rats supplied with restricted diet and having same pattern of weight loss resembling weight loss pattern observed in DM rats.

3.11. Expected mechanism of type 1 diabetes detrimental effects on tooth

Many investigations focused on the various detrimental effects exerted by the type 1 diabetes on different body organs; however, less attention was paid to the effect of such condition on teeth. A previous study suggested that the diabetic condition may exert detrimental effects on enamel formation [91]. However, that study was conducted on an extremely small sample size of different types of rodents suffering from diabetic conditions that were either genetically induced or drug induced and did not include a proper number of control rats. Thus, it was of an extreme importance to study the detrimental effect of diabetes on tooth structure formation using enough number of experimental animals and to use accurate methods of measurements as those adopted in the our studies. The null hypotheses tested in our previous study were partly accepted because the type 1 diabetes condition adversely affected the enamel and dentine thickness, and the dentine mineral apposition and dentine formation rates; however, there was no significant effect of the type 1 diabetes condition on the enamel and dentine mineral densities.

We have demonstrated that the type 1 diabetes condition induced detrimental changes on the thickness of enamel and dentine. Thus, it could be speculated that the metabolic functions of the ameloblasts and the odontoblasts may be hindered by the elevated blood glucose level associated with the type 1 diabetes condition. It was previously suggested that the type 1 diabetes condition affect ameloblasts and odontoblasts by a mechanism similar to the well-documented mechanism exerted by the type 1 diabetes condition on osteoblasts bone-forming cells due to the similarities between the process of dentine, enamel, and bone development [92]. Moreover, several genetic disorders were found to affect both the osteoblasts and odontoblasts and thus affecting the mineralization process of bone and dentine, respectively [92]. However, in contrast to bone, dentine and enamel do not remodel and are not involved in the regulation of the calcium and phosphate metabolism [93].

It was previously demonstrated that a glucose concentration similar to those observed in poorly controlled diabetic patients inhibited the osteoblast cells from depositing calcium during the mineralization process of the bone matrix [94]. One can speculate that a similar inhibitory effect was exhibited in the current study by the high glucose level on the activities of the odontoblasts and ameloblasts during the enamel and dentine formation. This inhibitory effect of increased glucose level on ameloblasts and odontoblasts was suggested by a previous study that showed that the total calcium content in rat teeth suffering from type 1 diabetes was significantly lower than those of their controls [95]. Another study reported a significant decrease in cultured pulp cells ability to proliferate and decreased mineralized nodule formation upon exposure to high levels of glucose [96]. Another mechanism that might explain the negative effects exerted by the type 1 diabetes condition on odontoblasts and ameloblasts activities may be attributed to the increase in blood glucose level that interferes with the maturation and the proper mineralization of the dentine collagen matrix during the dentine development stages [97]. Previous research work showed that the histological features of the ameloblast and its function might be affected by the increased glucose level associated with the type 1 diabetes condition [98]. Moreover, several clinical observations showed that enamel susceptibility to caries and the incidence of enamel hypoplasia increased in type 1 diabetes patients [99]. Furthermore, it was previously suggested that type 1 diabetes condition may exert a generalized decrease in the metabolic activities of bone cells. All of the aforementioned findings may suggest that the observed harmful effects exerted by the type 1 diabetes condition on enamel and dentine in this study may be a part of a generalized detrimental effect exerted by the diabetic condition on osteoblasts, odontoblasts, and ameloblasts.

4. Conclusion

It is obvious that type 1 diabetes condition significantly affects craniofacial growth, bone formation mechanism, and the quality of the bone formed, which may alter many aspects of planning and treatment of orthodontic patients affected by this globally increasing hormonal disturbance. Moreover, type 1 diabetes condition impairs the proper tooth development and alters the oral environment rendering teeth more susceptible to dental caries. There should be a new strategy for treating orthodontic patients suffering from metabolic disorders specially those disorders having direct and indirect effects on bone growth as the diabetic condition. The orthodontic craniofacial linear measurements were significantly decreased in the type 1 diabetes cases when compared to normal cases. Moreover, greater risks of developing dental caries and possible tooth loss are associated with patients suffering from type 1 diabetes; these risks may complicate the outcome of orthodontic treatment which is associated with less ability of orthodontic patients to implement proper oral hygiene measures due to increased areas of bacterial biofilm formation around orthodontic brackets. These comprehensive studies carried out on bone and craniofacial growth suggest that planning the treatment in craniofacial region for patients affected with hormonal disorders is more complex procedure than the treatment of normal patients. Up-to-date data also suggest that it is of prime importance to keep close attention to the general systemic condition of these patients and administer the proper hormonal therapy for these patients when needed to avoid any detrimental effects on bone resulting from any hormonal imbalance. Moreover, the results of tooth analysis in experimental type 1 diabetes model showed that the type 1 diabetes condition suppressed the enamel and dentine formation; however, the enamel and dentine densities were not affected. This indicates that diabetic patients may be more susceptible to dental caries and teeth size discrepancies. Type 1 diabetes patients' dental problems should be handled carefully, and their diabetic condition monitoring is of prime importance, especially during early stage of tooth development.

Author details

Ippei Watari[1*], Mona Aly Abbassy[2,3], Katarzyna Anna Podyma-Inoue[4] and Takashi Ono[1]

*Address all correspondence to: ippeiwatari@gmail.com

1 Orthodontic Science, Department of Orofacial Development and Function, Division of Oral Health Science, Graduate School of Medical and Dental Science, Tokyo Medical and Dental University (TMDU), Tokyo, Japan

2 Department of Orthodontics, Faculty of Dentistry, King Abdulaziz University, Jeddah, Saudi Arabia

3 Alexandria University, Alexandria, Egypt

4 Section of Biochemistry, Department of Bio-Matrix, Graduate School of Medical and Dental Science, Tokyo Medical and Dental University (TMDU), Tokyo, Japan

References

[1] Harjutsalo, V., Sjoberg, L., & Tuomilehto, J. (2008). Time trends in the incidence of type 1 diabetes in Finnish Children: a cohort study. *Lancet*, 371 (9626), 1777–1782.

[2] Onkamo, P., Vaananen, S., Karvonen, M., & Tuomilehto, J. (1999). Worldwide increase in incidence of type 1 diabetes—the analysis of the data on published incidence trends. *Diabetologia*, 42 (12), 1395–1403.

[3] WURODIAB ACE Study Group. (2000). Variation and trends in incidence of child-hood diabetes in Surope. *Lancet*, 355, 873–876.

[4] Guariguata, L. (2011). Estimating the worldwide burden of type 1 diabetes. *Diabetes Voice*, 56(2), 6–8.

[5] Zhukouskaya V, Eller-Vainicher C, Shepelkevich AP, Dydyshko Y, Cairoli E, Chiodi-ni I. (2015) Bone health in type 1 diabetes: focus on evaluation and treatment in clini-cal practice. Journal of Endocrinological Investigation 38(9) 941-950.

[6] Janghormani, M., van Dam, R. M., Willett W. C., & Hu, F. B. (2007). Systemic review of type 1 and type 2 diabetes mellitus and risk of fracture. *American Journal Epidemiology*, 166, 495–505.

[7] Vestergaard, P., (2007). Discrepancies in bone mineral density and fracture risk in pa-tients with type 1 and type 2 diabetes—a metanalysis. *Osteoporosis International*, 18, 427–444.

[8] Hamada, Y., Kitazawa, S., Kitazawa, R., Fujii, H., Kasuga, M., & Fukagawa, M. (2007). Histomorphometric analysis of diabetic osteopenia in streptozotocin-induced diabetic mice: a possible role of oxidative stress. *Bone*, 40(5), 1408–1418.

[9] Lu, H., Kraut D., Gerstenfeld, L. C., & Graves, D. T. (2003). Diabetes interferes with the bone formation by affecting the expression of transcription factors that regulate osteoblast differentiation. *Endocrinology*, 144(1), 346–352.

[10] Reddy, G. K., Stehno-Bittel, L., Hamade, S., & Enwemeka, C. S. (2001). The biome-chanical integrity of bone in experimental diabetes. *Diabetes Research Clinical Practice*, 54(1), 1–8.

[11] Ogata, N., Chikazu, D., Kubota, N., Terauchi, Y., Tobe, K., Azuma, Y., Ohta, T., Ka-dowaki, T., Nakamura, K., & Kawaguchi, H. (2000). Insulin receptor substrate-1 in osteoblast is indispensable for maintaining bone turnover. *Journal of Clinical Investigation*, 105 (7), 935–943.

[12] Albright, F., & Reifestein, E. C. (1948). Bone development in diabetic children: a roentgen study. *The American Journal of the Medical Sciences*, 174, 313–319.

[13] Levin, M. E., Boisseau, V. C., & Avioli, L. V. (1976). Effects of diabetes mellitus on bone mass in juvenile and adult onset diabetes. *The New England Journal of Medicine*, 294(5), 241–245.

[14] Munoz-Torres, M., Jodar, E., Escobar-Jimenez, F., López-Ibarra, P. J., & Luna, J. D. (1996). Bone mineral density measured by dual X-ray absorptiometry in Spanish pa-tients with insulin-dependent diabetes mellitus. *Calcified Tissue International*, 58 (5), 316–319.

[15] Miazgowski, T., & Czekalski, S. (1998). A 2-year follow-up study on bone mineral density and markers of bone turnover in patients with long-standing insulin-dependent diabetes mellitus. *Osteoporosis International*, 8(5), 399–403.

[16] Jehle, P. M., Jehle, E. R., Mohan, S., & Böhm, B. O. (1998). Serum levels of insulin-like growth factor system components and relationship to bone metabolism in type 1 and type 2 diabetes mellitus patients. *Journal of Endocrinology*, 159(2), 297–306.

[17] Tuominen, J. T., Impivaara, O., Puukka, P., & Rönnemaa, T. (1999). Bone mineral density in patients with type 1 and type 2 diabetes. *Diabetes Care*, 22(7), 1196–200.

[18] Gallacher, S. J., Fenner, J. A., Fischer, B. M., Quin, J. D., Fraser, W. D., Logue, F. C., Cowan, R. A., Boyle, I. T., & MacCuish, A. C. (1993). An evaluation of bone density and turnover in premenopausal women with type 1 diabetes mellitus. *Diabetic Medicine*, 10(2), 129–133.

[19] Weber, G., Beccaria, L., deAngelis, M., Mora, S., Galli, L., Cazzuffi, M., A., Turba, F., Frisone, F., Guarneri, M., P., & Chiumello, G. (1990). Bone mass in young patients with type 1 diabetes. *Bone and Mineral*, 8(1), 23–30.

[20] Pascual, J., Argente, J., & Lopezetal M. B. (1998). Bone mineral density in children and adolescents with diabetes mellitus type 1 of recent onset. *Calcified Tissue International*, 62(1), 31–35.

[21] Salvatoni, A., Mancassola, G., Biasoli, R., Cardani, R., Salvatore, S., Broggini· M., & Nespoli· L. (2004). Bone mineral density in diabetic children and adolescents: a follow-up study. *Bone*, 34(5), 900–904.

[22] Brandao, F. R., Vicente, E. J., Daltro, C. H., Sacramento, M., Moreira, A., & Adan, L. (2007). Bone metabolism is linked to disease duration and metabolic control in type 1 diabetes mellitus. *Diabetes Research and Clinical Practice*, 78(3), 334–339.

[23] Liu, E. Y., Wactawski-Wende, J., Donahue, R. P., Dmochowski, J., Hovey, K. M., & Quattrin T. (2003). Does low bone mineral density start in post-teenage years in women with type 1 diabetes? *Diabetes Care*, 26(8), 2365–2369.

[24] Mastrandrea, L. D., Wactawski-Wende, J., Donahue, R. P., Hovey, K. M., Clark, A., & Quattrin, T. (2008). Young women with type 1 diabetes have lower bone mineral density that persists over time. *Diabetes Care*, 31(9), 1729–1735.

[25] Bechtold, S., Dirlenbach, I., Raile, K., Noelle, V., Bonfig, W., & Schwarz, H. P. (2006). Early manifestation of type 1 diabetes in children is a risk factor for changed bone geometry: data using peripheral quantitative computed tomography. *Pediatrics*, 118(3), e627–e634.

[26] Maggio, A. B. R., Ferrari, S., & Kraenzlinetal, M. (2010). Decreased bone turnover in children and adolescents with well controlled type 1 diabetes. *Journal of Pediatric Endocrinology and Metabolism*, 23(7), 697–707.

[27] Gunczler, P., Lanes, R., Paz-Martinez, V., Martins, R., Esaa, S., Colmenares, V., & Weisinger, J., R. (1998). Decreased lumbar spine bone mass and low bone turnover in children and adolescents with insulin dependent diabetes mellitus followed longitudinally. *Journal of Pediatric Endocrinology and Metabolism*, 11(3), 413–419.

[28] Valerio, G., del Puente, A., Esposito-del Puente, A., Buono, P., Mozzillo, E., & Franzese, A. (2002). The lumbar bone mineral density is affected by long-term poor metabolic control in adolescents with type1 diabetes mellitus. *Hormone Research*, 58(6), 266–272.

[29] Heilman, K., Zilmer, M., Zilmer, K., & Tillmann, V. (2009). Lower bone mineral density in children with type 1 diabetes is associated with poor glycemic control and higher serum ICAM1 and urinary isoprostane levels. *Journal of Bone and Mineral Metabolism*, 27(5), 598–604.

[30] L'eger, J., Marinovic, D., Alberti, C., Dorgeret, S., Chevenne, D., Marchal, C. L., Tubiana-Rufi, N., Sebag, G., & Czernichow, P. (2006). Lower bone mineral content in children with type 1 diabetes mellitus is linked to female sex, low insulin-like growth factor type I levels, and high insulin requirement. *Journal of Clinical Endocrinology and Metabolism*, 91(10), 3947–3953.

[31] Saha, M. T. Sievänen, H., Salo, M., K. Tulokas, S., & Saha, H. H. (2009). Bone mass and structure in adolescents with type 1 diabetes compared to healthy peers. *Osteoporosis International*, 20(8), 1401–1406.

[32] Heap, J., Murray, M. A., Miller, S. C., Jalili, T., & Moyer Mileur, L. J. (2004). Alterations in bone characteristics associated with glycemic control in adolescents with type 1 diabetes mellitus. *Journal of Pediatrics*, 144(1), 56–62.

[33] Hamed, E. A., Abu Faddan, N. H., Adb Elhafeez, H. A., & Sayed, D. (2011). Parathormone—25(OH)-vitamin D axis and bone status in children and adolescents with type1 diabetes mellitus. *Pediatric Diabetes*, 12(6), 536–546.

[34] Liu, E. Y., Wactawski-Wende, J., Donahue, R. P., Dmochowski, J., Hovey, K. M., & Quattrin, T. (2003). Does low bone mineral density start in post-teenage years in women with type 1 diabetes? *Diabetes Care*, 26(8), 2365–2389.

[35] Mastrandrea, L. D., Wactawski-Wenda, J., Donahue, R. P., Hovey, K. M., Clark, A., & Quattrin, T. (2008). Young women with type 1 diabetes have lower bone mineral density that persists over time. *Diabetes Care*, 31(9), 1729–1735.

[36] Kemink, S. A. G., Hermus, A. R. M. M., Swinkels, L. M. J. W., Lutterman, J. A., & Smals, A. G. H. (2000). Osteopenia in insulin-dependent diabetes mellitus: prevalence and aspects of pathophysiology. *Journal of Endocrinology Investigation*, 23(5), 295–303.

[37] Rozasilla, A., Nolla, J. M., Montana, E., Fiter, J., Gomez-Vaquero, C., Soler, J., & Roig-Escofet, D. (2000). Bone mineral density in patients with type 1 diabetes mellitus. *Joint Bone Spine*, 67(3), 215–218.

[38] Hadjidakis, D. J., Raptis, A. E., Sfakianakis, M., Mylonakis, A., & Raptis, S. A. (2006). Bone mineral density of both genders in type 1 diabetes according to bone composition. *Journal of Diabetes and its Complications*, 20(5), 302–307.

[39] Danielson, K. K., Elliott, M. E., Lecaire, T., Binkley, N., & Palta, M. (2009). Poor glycemic control is associated with low BMD detected in premenopausal women with type 1 diabetes. *Osteoporosis International*, 20(6), 923–933.

[40] Alexopoulou, O., Jamart, J., Devogelaer, J. P., Brichard, S. de Nayer, P., & Buyysschaert, M. (2006). Bone density and markers of bone remodeling in type 1 male diabetic patients. *Diabetes and Metabolism*, 32(5), 453–458.

[41] Hampson, G., Evans, C., Petttit, R. J., Evans, W. D., Woodhead, S. J., Peters, J. R., & Ralston, S. H. (1998). Bone mineral density, collagen type 1 alpha 1 genotypes and bone turnover in premenopausal women with diabetes mellitus. *Diabetologia*, 41(11), 1314–1320.

[42] Ingberg, C. M., Palmer, M., Aman, J., Arvidsson, B., Schvarcz, E., & Berne, C. (2004). Body composition and bone mineral density in long-standing type 1 diabetes. *Journal of International Medicine*, 255(3), 392–398.

[43] Bridges, M. J., Moochhala, S. H., Barbour, J., & Kelly, C. A. (2005). Influence of diabetes on peripheral bone mineral density in men: a controlled study. *Acta Diabetologica*, 42(2), 82–86.

[44] Vestergaard, P. (2007). Discrepancies in bone mineral density and fracture risk in patients with type 1 and type 2 diabetes—a meta-analysis. *Osteoporosis International*, 18(4), 427–444.

[45] Zhukouskaya V. V., Eller-Vainicher C., Vadzianava V. V., Shepelkevich A. P., Zhurava I. V., Korolenko G. G., Salko O. B., Cairoli E., Beck-Peccoz P., Chiodini I. (2013) Prevalence of morphometric vertebral fractures in patients with type 1 diabetes. Diabetes Care, 36(6):1635-40.

[46] Inoue, Y., Hisa, I., Seino, S., & Kaji, H. (2010). Alendronate induces mineralization in mouse osteoblastic MC3T3-E1 cells: regulation of mineralization-related genes. *Experimental Clinical Endocrinology and Diabetes*, 118(10), 719–723.

[47] Aoyama, E., Watari, I., Podyma-Inoue, K. A., Yanagishita, M., & Ono, T. (2014). Expression of glucagon-like peptide-1 receptor and glucose-dependent insulinotropic polypeptide receptor is regulated by the glucose concentration in mouse osteoblastic MC3T3-E1 cells. *International Journal of Molecular Medicine*, 34(2), 475–478.

[48] Baggio, L. L., & Drucker, D. J. (2007). Biology of incretins: GLP-1 and GIP. *Gastroenterology*, 132(6), 2131–2157.

[49] Yamada, C., Yamada, Y., Tsukiyama, K., Yamada, K., Udagawa, N., Takahashi, N., Tanaka, K., Drucker, D. J., Seino, Y., & Inagaki, N. (2008). The murine glucagon-like peptide-1 receptor is essential for control of bone resorption. *Endocrinology*, 149(2), 574–579.

[50] Driessen, J. H., van Onzenoort, H. A., Henry, R. M., Lalmohamed, A., van den Bergh, J. P., Neef, C., Leufkens, H. G., & de Vries, F. (2014). Use of dipeptidyl peptidase-4 inhibitors for type 2 diabetes mellitus and risk of fracture. *Bone*, 68, 124–130.

[51] Bensch, L., Braem, M., Van Acker, K., & Willems, G. (2003). Orthodontic treatment considerations in patients with diabetes mellitus. *American Journal of Orthodontics and Dentofacial Orthopedics*, 123(1), 74–78.

[52] Giglio, M. J., & Lama, M. A. (2001). Effect of experimental diabetes on mandible growth in rats. *European Journal of Oral Sciences*, 109(3), 193–197.

[53] Salzmann, J. A. (1979). Practice of orthodontics under public health guidance. *American Journal of Orthodontics*, 76(1), 103–104.

[54] Kumar, P., & Clark, M. (2009). Kumar and Clark's Clinical Medicine (7th edition), Elsevier.

[55] El-Bialy, T., Aboul-Azm, S. F., & El-Sakhawy, M. (2000). Study of craniofacial morphology and skeletal maturation in juvenile diabetics (type I). *American Journal of Orthodontics and Dentofacial Orthopedics*, 118(2), 189–195.

[56] Roe, T. F., Mora, S., Costen, G., Kaufman, F., Carlson, M., & Gilsanz, V. (1991). Vertebral bone density in insulin-dependent diabetic children. *Metabolism*, 40(9), 967–971.

[57] Abbassy, M. A., Watari, I., & Soma, K. (2008). Effect of experimental diabetes on craniofacial growth in rats. *Archives of Oral Biology*, 53(9), 819–825.

[58] Hough, S., Avioli, L. V., Bergfeld, M. A., Fallon, M. D., Slatopolsky, E., & Teitelbaum, S. L. (1981). Correction of abnormal bone and mineral metabolism in chronic streptozotocin-induced diabetes mellitus in the rat by insulin therapy. *Endocrinology*, 108(6), 2228–2234.

[59] Tein, MS, Breen, S. A., Loveday, B. E., Devlin, H., Balment, R. J., Boyd, R. D., Sibley CP, Garland HO.. (1998). Bone mineral density and composition in rat pregnancy: effects of streptozotocin-induced diabetes mellitus and insulin replacement. *Experimental Physiology*, 83(2), 165–174.

[60] Thrailkill, K. M., Liu, L., Wahl, E. C., Bunn, R. C., Perrien, D. S., Cockrell, G. E., Skinner RA, Hogue WR, Carver AA, Fowlkes JL, Aronson J, Lumpkin CK Jr. (2005). Bone formation is impaired in a model of type 1 diabetes. *Diabetes*, 54(10), 2875–2881.

[61] Follak, N., Kloting, I., Wolf, E., & Merk, H. (2004). Histomorphometric evaluation of the influence of the diabetic metabolic state on bone defect healing depending on the defect size in spontaneously diabetic BB/OK rats. *Bone*, 35(1), 144–152.

[62] Alkan, A., Erdem, E., Gunhan, O., & Karasu, C. (2002). Histomorphometric evaluation of the effect of doxycycline on the healing of bone defects in experimental diabetes mellitus: a pilot study. *Journal of Oral and Maxillofacial Surgery*, 60(8), 898–904.

[63] Mc Cracken-Wesson, M. S., Aponte, R., Chavali, R., & Lemons, J. E. (2006). Bone associated with implants in diabetic and insulin-treated rats. *Clinical Oral Implants Research*, 17(5), 495–500.

[64] Abdus, Salam. M., Matsumoto, N., Matin, K., Tsuha, Y., Nakao, R., Hanada, N., & Senpuku, H. (2004). Establishment of an animal model using recombinant NOD.B10.D2 mice to study initial adhesion of oral streptococci. *Clinical and Diagnostic Laboratory Immunology*, 11(2), 379–386.

[65] Matin, K., Salam, M. A., Akhter, J., Hanada, N., & Senpuku, H. (2002). Role of stromal-cell derived factor-1 in the development of autoimmune diseases in non-obese diabetic mice. *Immunology*, 107(2), 222–232.

[66] Chidiac, J. J., Shofer, F. S., Al-Kutoub, A., Laster, L. L., & Ghafari, J. (2002). Comparison of CT scanograms and cephalometric radiographs in craniofacial imaging. *Orthodontics and Craniofacial Research*, 5(2), 104–113.

[67] Vande Berg, J. R., Buschang, P. H., & Hinton, R. J. (2004). Absolute and relative growth of the rat craniofacial skeleton. *Archives of Oral Biology*, 49(6), 477–484.

[68] Engstrom, C., Jennings, J., Lundy, M., & Baylink, D. J. (1988). Effect of bone matrix-derived growth factors on skull and tibia in the growing rat. *Journal of Oral Pathology*, 17(7), 334–340.

[69] Kiliaridis, S. E. C., & Thilander, B. (1985). The relationship between masticatory function and craniofacial morphology. I. A cephalometric longitudinal analysis in the growing rat fed a soft diet. *European Journal of Orthodontics*, 7, 273–283.

[70] Vandeberg, J. R., Buschang, P. H., & Hinton, R. J. (2004). Craniofacial growth in growth hormone-deficient rats. The anatomical record. Part A. *Discoveries in Molecular, Cellular and Evolutionary Biology*, 278(2), 561–570.

[71] Stuart, A., & Smith, D. (1992). Use of the fluorochromes xylenol orange, calcein green, and tetracycline to document bone deposition and remodeling in healing fractures in chickens. *Avian Diseases*, 36 (2), 447–449.

[72] Abbassy, M. A., Watari, I., & Soma, K. (2010). The effect of diabetes mellitus on rat mandibular bone formation and microarchitecture. *European Journal of Oral Sciences*, 118(4), 364–369.

[73] Shimomoto, Y., Chung, C. J., Iwasaki-Hayashi, Y., Muramoto, T., & Soma, K. (2007). Effects of occlusal stimuli on alveolar/jaw bone formation. *Journal of Dental Research*, 86(1), 47–51.

[74] Parfitt, A. M. (1988). Bone histomorphometry: standardization of nomenclature, symbols and units (summary of proposed system). *Bone*, 9(1), 67–69.

[75] Keshawarz, N. M., & Recker, R. R. (1986). The label escape error: comparison of measured and theoretical fraction of total bone-trabecular surface covered by single label in normals and patients with osteoporosis. *Bone*, 7(2), 83–87.

[76] Sheng, M. H., Baylink, D. J., Beamer, W. G., Donahue, L. R., Rosen, C. J., Lau, K. H., Wergedal JE. (1999). Histomorphometric studies show that bone formation and bone mineral apposition rates are greater in C3H/HeJ (high-density) than C57BL/6J (low-density) mice during growth. *Bone*, 25(4), 421–429.

[77] Gerlach, R. F., Toledo, D. B., Fonseca, R. B., Novaes, P. D., Line, S. R., & Merzel, J. (2002). Alveolar bone remodelling pattern of the rat incisor under different functional conditions as shown by minocycline administration. *Archives of Oral Biology*, 47(3), 203–209.

[78] Siudikiene, J., Machiulskiene, V., Nyvad, B., Tenovuo, J., & Nedzelskiene, I. (2006). Dental caries and salivary status in children with type 1 diabetes mellitus, related to the metabolic control of the disease. *European Journal of Oral Sciences*, 114(1), 8–14.

[79] Abbassy, M. A., Watari, I., Barkry, A. S., Hamba, H., Hassan, A. H., Tagami, T., & Ono, T. (2015). Diabetes detrimental effects on enamel and dentin formation. *Journal of Dentistry*, 43(5), 589–596.

[80] Losken, A., Mooney, M. P., & Siegel, M. I. (1994). Comparative cephalometric study of nasal cavity growth patterns in seven animal models. *Cleft Palate Craniofacial Journal*, 31(1), 17–23.

[81] Siegel, M. I., & Mooney, M. P. (1990). Appropriate animal models for craniofacial biology. *Cleft Palate Journal*, 27(1), 18–25.

[82] Duarte, V. M., Ramos, A. M., Rezende, L. A., Macedo, U. B., Brandao-Neto, J., Almeida, M. G., & Rezende, A. A. (2005). Osteopenia: a bone disorder associated with diabetes mellitus. *Journal of Bone and Mineral Metabolism*, 23(1), 58–68.

[83] Ward, D. T., Yau, S. K., Mee, A. P., Mawer, E. B., Miller, CA, Garland, H. O., et al. (2001). Functional, molecular, and biochemical characterization of streptozotocin-induced diabetes. *Journal of the American Society of Nephrology*, 12(4), 779–790.

[84] Pun, K. K., Lau, P., & Ho, P. W. (1989). The characterization, regulation, and function of insulin receptors on osteoblast-like clonal osteosarcoma cell line. *Journal of Bone and Mineral Research*, 4(6), 853–862.

[85] Thomas, D. M., Udagawa, N., Hards, D. K., Quinn, J. M., Moseley, J. M., Findlay, D. M., Best JD. (1998). Insulin receptor expression in primary and cultured osteoclast-like cells. *Bone*, 23(3), 181–186

[86] Reddy, G. K., Stehno-Bittel, L., Hamade, S., & Enwemeka, C. S. (2001). The biome-chanical integrity of bone in experimental diabetes. *Diabetes Research and Clinical Prac-tice*, 54(1), 1–8.

[87] Tsuchida, T., Sato, K., Miyakoshi, N., Abe, T., Kudo, T., Tamura, Y., Kasukawa Y, Su-zuki K. (2000). Histomorphometric evaluation of the recovering effect of human par-athyroid hormone (1–34) on bone structure and turnover in streptozotocin-induced diabetic rats. *Calcified Tissue International*, 66(3), 229–233.

[88] Toromanoff, A., Ammann, P., Mosekilde, L., Thomsen, J. S., & Riond, J. L. (1997). Par-athyroid hormone increases bone formation and improves mineral balance in vita-min D-deficient female rats. *Endocrinology*, 138(6), 2449–2457.

[89] Collins, D., Jasani, C., Fogelman, I., & Swaminathan, R. (1998). Vitamin D and bone mineral density. *Osteoporosis International*, 8(2), 110–114.

[90] Chiarelli, F., Giannini, C., & Mohn, A. (2004). Growth, growth factors and diabetes. *European Journal of Endocrinology*, 151(3), U109–U117.

[91] Atar, M., Atar-Zwillenberg, D. R., Verry, P., & Spornitz, U. M. (2004). Defective en-amel ultrastructure in diabetic rodents. *International Journal of Paediatric Dentistry*, 14, 301–307.

[92] Opsahl Vital, S., Gaucher, C., Bardet, C., Rowe, P. S., George, A., Linglart, A., & Chaussain, C. (2012). Tooth dentin defects reflect genetic disorders affecting bone mineralization. *Bone*, 50(4), 989–997.

[93] Chen, S., Rani, S., Wu, Y., Unterbrink, A., Gu, T. T., Gluhak-Heinrich, J, Chuang, H. H., & Macdougall, M. (2005). Differential regulation of dentin sialophosphoprotein expression by Runx2 during odontoblast cytodifferentiation. *The Journal of Biological Chemistry*, 280(33), 29717–29727.

[94] Balint, E., Szabo, P., Marshall, C. F., & Sprague, S. M. (2001). Glucose-induced inhibi-tion of in vitro bone mineralization. *Bone*, 28 (1), 21–28.

[95] Gutowska, I., Baranowska-Bosiacka, I., Rybicka, M., Nocen, I., Dudzinska, W., Marchlewicz, M., Wiszniewska, B., & Chlubek, D. (2011). Changes in the concentra-tion of microelements in the teeth of rats in the final stage of type 1 diabetes, with an absolute lack of insulin. *Biology of Trace Element Research*, 139(3), 332–340.

[96] Yeh, C. K., Harris, S. E., Mohan, S., Horn, D., Fajardo, R., Chun, Y. H., Jorgensen, J., Macdougall, M., & Abboud-Werner, S. (2012). Hyperglycemia and xerostomia are key determinants of tooth decay in type 1 diabetic mice. *Laboratory Investigation*, 92, 868–882.

[97] Valikangas, L., Pekkala, E., Larmas, M., Risteli, J., Salo, T., & Tjaderhane, L. (2001). The effects of high levels of glucose and insulin on type I collagen synthesis in ma-ture human odontoblasts and pulp tissue in vitro. *Advances in Dental Research*, 15, 72–75.

[98] Silva-Sousa, Y. T., Peres, L. C., & Foss, M. C. (2003). Are there structural alterations in the enamel organ of offspring of rats with alloxan-induced diabetes mellitus? *Brazilian Dental Journal*, 14(3), 162–167.

[99] Siudikiene, J., Machiulskiene, V., Nyvad, B., Tenovuo, J., & Nedzelskiene, I. (2008). Dental caries increments and related factors in children with type 1 diabetes mellitus. *Caries Research*, 42(5), 354–362.

6

The Innate Immune System via Toll-Like Receptors (TLRs) in Type 1 Diabetes - Mechanistic Insights

Kenia Pedrosa Nunes, Eric Guisbert, Theodora Szasz and Clinton Webb

Abstract

Type 1 diabetes (T1D) is a form of diabetes mellitus resulting from the lack of insulin secretion by the pancreatic beta cells and which accounts for approximately 5% of the total number of patients with diabetes worldwide. T1D is one of the most common endocrine disorders of children, and its incidence is steadily increasing. T1D is largely considered an autoimmune disorder resulting from the specific destruction of the pancreatic beta-cells that produce insulin. However, T1D pathophysiology is still not completely understood, and although insulin and other therapies ameliorate the manifestations of the disease, no cure is currently available. Traditionally, T1D has been thought of as a condition of cellular adaptive immunity, but evidence exists that components of the innate immune system, such as Toll-like receptors (TLRs), play a critical role in T1D development. TLRs have a central role in sensing microbial infections as well as endogenous alarm signals and trigger the release of inflammatory cytokines. The involvement of these receptors in the pathophysiology of several chronic diseases has become a major research interest, and in the last two decades, many studies have suggested the involvement of the innate immune system in the mechanism triggering T1D. Furthermore, microvascular complications in diabetic patients result in considerable morbidity, particularly diabetic nephropathy, retinopathy, and atherosclerosis. A hallmark of diabetic vascular pathology is inflammation and endothelial dysfunction. Recent literature suggests that TLR signaling is involved in vascular inflammation and endothelial dysfunction and that TLR activation may play a crucial role in diabetic microangiopathy. However, the mechanisms by which TLRs and their ligands contribute to T1D are not yet clear, and further investigation is needed. The goal of the present chapter is to address the contribution of TLRs to the mechanisms leading to the development and progression of T1D and to review current possibilities of targeting TLRs to forestall diabetic complications.

Keywords: Toll-like receptors, type 1 diabetes, DAMPS, innate immune system, microangiopathy

1. Introduction

The innate immune system is the first line of defense against invading organisms and other dangerous events in our body. Unlike the acquired immune system, innate immunity identifies the presence of harm via pattern recognition receptors (PRRs). Toll-like receptors (TLRs) are one of the most important classes of PRRs for sensing harmful signals. TLRs can recognize two types of molecules: (1) conserved pathogen molecules such as lipopolysaccharide (LPS), proteins, and nucleic acids expressed by microbes, viruses, bacteria, and fungi, which are known as pathogen-associated molecular patterns or PAMPS [1-2] and (2) endogenous molecules released from damaged cells or tissues such as HMGB-1, HSP60, and C-reactive protein called damage-associated patterns or DAMPS [3]. To date, ten TLRs have been identified in humans (TLR1–TLR10) and twelve in mice (TLR1–TLR9 and TLR11–TLR13). Most TLRs are located on the cell surface, except for TLR3, TLR7, TLR8, and TLR9, which are expressed in the intracellular compartment, the endosome [4].

All TLRs share their intracellular domain with the interleukin-1-receptor (IL-1R) family. Two major intracellular signaling pathways are triggered by TLRs, one that is canonical and dependent on myeloid differentiation primary response protein 88 (MyD88) and another that is noncanonical and MyD88-independent (Figure 1) pathway. MyD88 binds to TLRs upon activation and is essential for the induction of inflammatory cytokines via TLRs. All TLRs, except TLR3, can activate a MyD88-dependent pathway, which involves mitogen-activated kinases and leads to the transcription of pro-inflammatory genes through the activation of nuclear factor κB (NF-κB). TLR3 activates the TRIF-mediated pathway, a MyD88-independent pathway that in turn activates interferon regulatory factor 3 (IRF-3), inducing the expression of interferons (IFNs) [5]. TLR pathway activation results in the activation of the inhibitor of NF-κB kinase (IKK) complex and the transcription factor nuclear factor κB (NF-κB). NF-κB has been extensively studied as a regulator of inflammatory mediators, including tumor necrosis factor alpha (TNF-α). Increased levels of interleukin 1 beta (IL-1β) and TNF-α have been correlated with an expression of TLR2 and TLR4 on monocytes from T1D patients [6] (Figure 1).

Type 1 diabetes (T1D) is a disease in which the pancreatic insulin-producing beta-cells are lost or destroyed, usually via autoimmune mechanisms. Consequently, slow and progressive islet beta-cell impairment and total loss of insulin secretion are observed [7-8]. How the disease is triggered is unknown; however, research in animal models of T1D supports the hypothesis that microbial infection and/or innate immune system activation play an important role in disease mechanisms [9]. Several lines of evidence suggest that T1D progression is strongly heritable [10-11]. However, in addition to genetic factors, environmental factors such as chemicals, infections, and components of early childhood diet might contribute to T1D onset [12]. The development of T1D can be classified into two stages. In the first stage, called insulitis, Langerhans islets in the pancreas are progressively infiltrated by cells of the immune system, especially T cells and macrophages (Figure 2). In the second stage, most beta-cells are destroyed by the infiltrating immune cells. Apoptosis of pancreatic beta-cells is the last step in the initial pathogenesis of T1D [13]. Regardless of the progress toward the last step of T1D development,

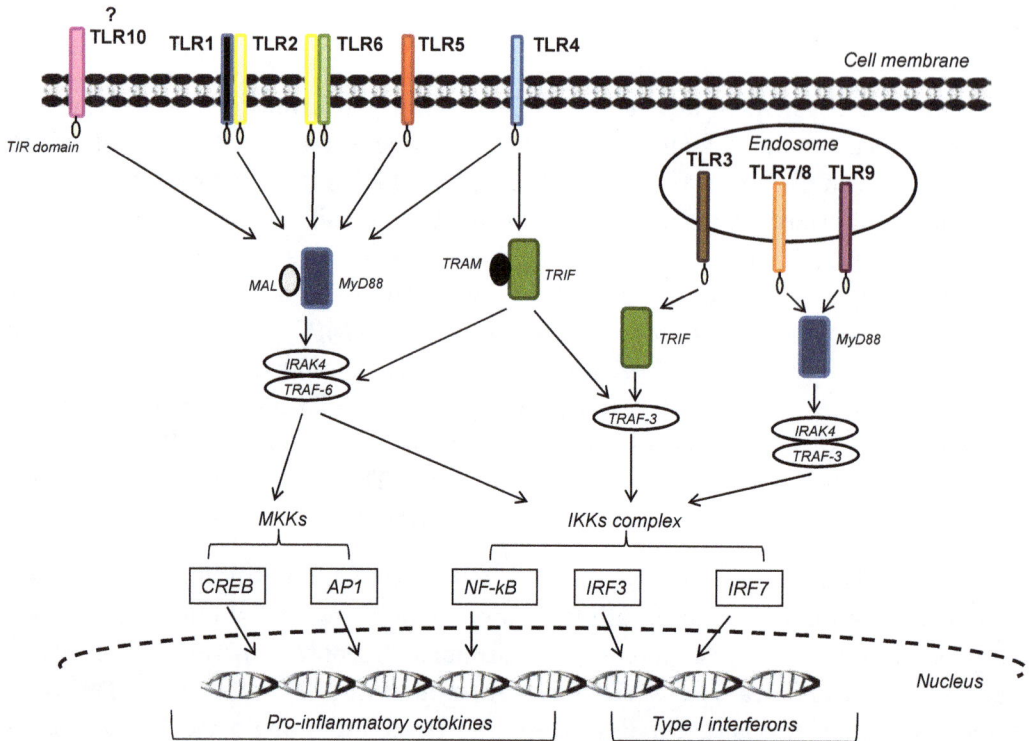

Figure 1. Ten human TLRs and their pathways. Signaling pathways activated by TLRs might be MyD88 dependent or independent. MyD88 is an adaptor molecule, which recruits IRAK and induces phosphorylation. IRAK associates with TRAF6 or TRAF3, leading to the activation of IKK complex or MKKs and resulting in the activation of NF-κB and other important transcription factors (CREB and AP1). The activation of a MyD88-dependent pathway leads to induction of inflammatory cytokines or type I interferons (IFNs). All TLRs, except TLR3, can activate MyD88. The MyD88-independent pathway is called TRIF-mediated pathway (TIR-domain-containing adaptor inducing an NF-κB). TLR4 can also utilize the TRIF-related adaptor molecule (TRAM) for the activation of NF-κB. In order to switch signaling from MyD88 to TRIF, TLR4 moves from plasma membrane to the endosomes. Little is known about TLR10 and its ligands, but this receptor may heterodimerize with TLR1 and TLR2. The activation of TLRs especially TLR2 and TLR4 pathways leads to complications that are associated with the pathogenesis of diabetes. CRBE: cyclic AMP-responsive element binding-protein; AP1: activator protein 1.

the initial step, triggering anti-islet autoimmunity, is still unclear and this is one of the most relevant issues in the field of autoimmune diseases.

Generally, TLR-expressing innate immune cells trigger the initial actions against dangerous signals, which later lead to the activation of T and B cells of the adaptive immune system. Although the primary function of TLRs is linked to the innate immunity, there are no reasons why TLRs may not have a direct function on adaptive immunity, and it has been recently demonstrated that TLRs are also expressed not only in cells from the innate immune but also in T and B cells [14-16]. Continuous release of DAMPs from damaged cells and tissues may maintain the activation of the innate immune system in diseases with long-term low-level inflammation. Therefore, the participation of innate immunity via TLRs not only in acute but also in chronic disease has been recently speculated in the literature. The expression of TLRs in T or B cells has been suggested to provide a cell intrinsic mechanism for innate signals

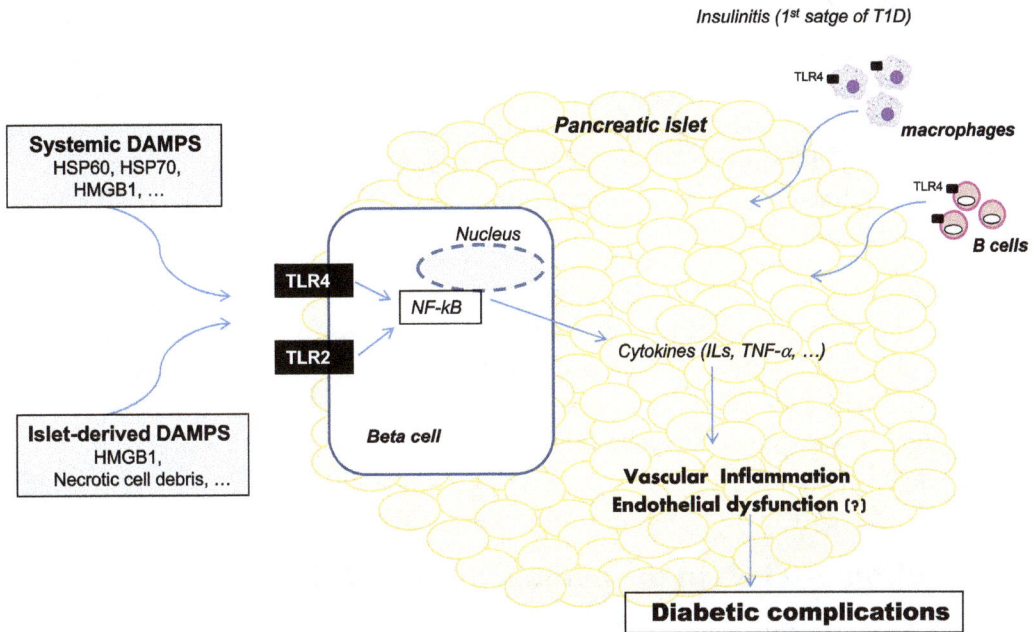

Figure 2. Involvement of TLR2 and TLR4 in the development of T1D. TLR2 and TLR4 on islet beta-cells senses expression changes in DAMPS such as HMGB1 and contribute to the initiation of T1D. Activation of TLR2 and TLR4 leads to NF-κB activation and pro-inflammatory cytokines production, which play a part in T1D inflammatory process and possibly endothelial dysfunction resulting in diabetic vascular complications. In addition, in T1D, the pancreas is progressively infiltrated by cells of the immune system such as macrophages and B-cells which express TLR2 and TLR4.

regulating adaptive immune responses [3, 16], which suggest the TLR-mediated activation of innate immunity may be controlling chronic disorders. However, the exact role of the innate immunity and TLRs in chronic diseases such as T1D is still under discussion.

TLRs play a major role in the development of several pancreatic diseases [17]. In the last decade, the involvement of the innate immune system in diabetes development and complications has been highlighted and investigated by many authors [18-19]. The idea that the initial event in the pathogenesis of autoimmune T1D comprises sensing of molecular patterns from apoptotic beta cells by TLRs has been suggested in recent papers [8, 20]. In T1D, necrotic beta-cells might stimulate dendritic cells (DCs), which are essential in defending against microbial infections and are involved in initiating and regulating immune responses linked to inflammation [21]. In addition, during the development of T1D, multiple interactions occur between DCs, macrophages, natural killer cells (NKs), and lymphocytes. Ultimately, the activation of these cells leads to induction of inflammatory genes [22]. A proinflammatory state is characteristic of T1D and is manifested by elevated circulating and cellular biomarkers such as augmented plasma levels of C-reactive proteins (CRP), cytokines (IL-1B, TNF, and IL-6), soluble cell protein adhesion, chemokines, etc. These increases are further accentuated in T1D patients with vascular complications [23-24].

Of the various TLRs, TLR2 and TLR4 have an important role in inflammation associated with diabetes. In addition, T1D harbors a considerably elevated risk for progressive atherosclerotic events and TLRs may be involved, but the mechanistic basis for this phenomenon is not completely clear. Likewise, TLRs are involved in the pathogenesis of diabetic microvascular alterations [25]. However, the TLR activation in this diabetic condition and its association with vascular or endothelial dysfunction has not been well characterized. Experimental studies have shown that TLR2 and TLR4 could be important participants in the progression of atherosclerosis in diabetes [6, 26-27]. On the other hand, TLR3, TLR7, and TLR9 seem to be involved in the initiation of TD1 [5, 28].

In this chapter, based on the recent advances in understanding the role of the innate immune system in chronic disease, we focus on the contribution of TLRs to the mechanisms that trigger T1D onset and the development of its complications. This information might provide new insights into possibilities for therapeutic intervention by targeting and modulating the immune system to abrogate or prevent T1D.

2. Contribution of TLRs in the pathogenesis of T1D

Recently, it has become evident that the dysregulation of the innate immune system can precipitate autoimmune diseases, including T1D. Given its essential role in orchestrating innate immune responses, the TLRs may be expected to play a significant role in the T1D development, progression, and its complications. The connections among inflammation, hyperglycemia, and diabetes have clear implications for the immune system. In addition, TLRs activate two types of downstream signaling pathways that lead to the activation of NF-κB with concomitant increase in inflammatory cytokine secretion (Figure 1). Both pathways contribute significantly to the pathophysiology of inflammation in endothelial dysfunction and are relevant to diabetic microangiopathy. Therefore, the key point regarding the involvement of TLRs in T1D and its complications seems to be the inflammatory process.

2.1. TLR2 and TLR4

The activation of the innate immune system via TLRs, in particular, TLR2 and TLR4, seems to play an important role in the development of T1D. Many authors proposed the sensing of DAMPs released from damaged pancreatic β-cells by TLR2 to be first event in the development of T1D [29-30]. The Increased expression of TLR2 and TLR4 in monocytes was described in patients with T1D compared to healthy patients [6]. In addition, the expression of TLR2 is augmented in T1D in both rat and human kidneys and has been associated with vascular complications [31]. Furthermore, T1D patients with microvascular complications showed increases in TLR2 and TLR4 activity in monocytes compared with matched controls [25]. The higher expression of TLR2 and TLR4 is associated with poor glycemic control, while the knockdown of both TLR2 and TLR4 resulted in a 76% decrease in a high glucose-induced NF-κB response, suggesting an additive effect [32-33]. Also, it has been demonstrated that deletion of TLR2 in mice significantly abrogates the proinflammatory state of T1D for up to 14 weeks in mice and improves the wound healing process, supporting a role for TLR2 in promoting inflammation in diabetes [30, 34].

There are ample data supporting an important role for inflammation associated with atherosclerosis in T1D and TLRs may be mediating this process. A recent study demonstrated that TLR2 and TLR4 mediate inflammatory pathways in endothelial cells exposed to high glucose [35], although the precise mechanism by which glucose fluctuations mediate inflammation in endothelial dysfunction is unknown. In apolipoprotein $E^{-/-}$ mice, the deficiency of IP-10 (interferon-gamma-inducible-protein 10) or its receptor (CXCR3) reduces vascular lesion formation. Also, elevated serum IP-10 levels have been shown in diabetes as well as increased monocytic IP-10 in T1D patients, but it is unclear if the patients had complications [36]. TLR4 agonists such as LPS have been shown to induce IP-10 production, and it has been demonstrated that down-regulation of TLR2 and TLR4 abrogates high glucose-induced IP-10 release via NF-κB inhibition [32].

Although many studies have highlighted the involvement of TLRs in the pathogenesis of T1D, TLRs might also have a beneficial role against T1D. Since the cause of T1D and the mechanisms involving this condition are not completely elucidated, the contradiction about the role of the TLRs in T1D could be dependent on the disease stage or how the disease was triggered. T cells, especially CD4 and CD25 T cells, play an important role in the prevention of autoimmunity. These cells not only express different TLRs, including TLR2, but are also functionally regulated directly or indirectly through TLR signaling [37-38]. Recently, it was showed that treatment of prediabetic mice with a synthetic TLR2 agonist diminished T1D and increased the number and function of CD4 and CD25 T cells, also conferring DCs with tolerogenic properties, suggesting that TLR2 signaling improves immunoregulation to prevent T1D [39]. On the other hand, another study suggested that TLR2 and MyD88 was dispensable for development of T1D in non obese diabetic (NOD) mice [40], which exhibit a susceptibility to spontaneous development of autoimmune insulin-dependent diabetes mellitus. NOD mice are a well established model of autoimmune diseases, including human T1D [41]. These data contrast with other reports showing the involvement of TLR2 in the initiation of autoimmune responses directed against beta-cells [42].

In NOD mice, the deletion of TLR4 results in acceleration of diabetes onset and immune cell infiltration of islets [43]. A recent study in the same animal model showed that TLR4 mediates cardiac lipid accumulation and diabetic heart disease [44]. On the contrary, treatment with a TLR4/MD-2 specific agonist monoclonal antibody (UT18) in NOD mice not only prevented T1D but also reversed new T1D onset diagnosed by polyuria, weight loss, and elevated blood glucose [45]. Supporting these results, an agonistic monoclonal antibody to TLR4/MD-2 reverses the development of diabetes in a high percentage of NOD mice. TLR4 antibody treatment increases T regulatory cell numbers in both the periphery and the pancreatic islet, suggesting a novel immunological tool for management of T1D in humans [46]. Taken together, these observations suggest a potential role for TLR2 and TLR4 in the pathology of diabetes. However, the mechanistic details need to be better investigated. Undoubtedly, the majority of existing data suggest that TLRs play a part in T1D, mediating T1D development and its complications, even if it is not clear if this is a beneficial role, a detrimental role, or a combination of the two.

2.2. Other TLRs and T1D

The role of the TLR pathway in the mechanism of T1D has been intensely investigated in the last decade, and it is undeniable that these receptors are involved in the pathogenesis of T1D. However, the majority of the studies are focused on TLR2 and TLR4 and only a few studies have discussed other TLRs such as TLR1, TLR3, TLR7, and TLR9.

To the best of our knowledge, there is only one study showing that TLR1 may be involved in the mechanism of diabetes. In this work, a detailed phenotypic analysis of the diabetes-resistant NOD.C3H-congenic strain 6 was evaluated, and the results suggested that TLR1 pathway is involved in the inflammatory response and the development of T1D controlled by the Idd6 locus [47].

The TLR3 gene codes for an endoplasmic receptor that recognizes dsRNA and plays an important role in the innate immune response initiated by viral infection. Although there are only a few studies reporting a link between T1D and TLR3 gene alterations, polymorphisms in the TLR3 gene seem to be linked to the risk of T1D. In fact, rs5743313 and rs117221827 polymorphisms were associated with an early age at diagnosis and worse glycemic control [48]. However, genotypic data on a small population of South Africans of Zulu origin suggested a weak association of the TLR3 polymorphism C2593T, C2642A, and A2690G with T1D [49]. The hypothesis that viral infections are involved in T1D is based on epidemiological studies [50]. One of the major observations that support a role for a viral etiology of T1D is that in accordance rates for T1D in monozygotic twins are only 50% instead of the expected 100% if the characteristic would be explained only by genetic factors. TLR3 is expressed at high levels in human and mouse pancreatic beta-cells and antigen-presenting DCs, and this receptor activates the TRIF-mediated pathway, which in turn activates interferon regulatory factor (IRF)-3 inducing the expression of IFNs. However, NF-κB may also be activated by TLR3 to upregulate the production of proinflammatory cytokines [5].

TLR7 stimulation activates DCs and T cells to promote autoimmune diabetes in nonobese diabetic (NOD) mice. Treatment with IRS661, an antagonist for TLR7, inhibits the activation of DCs and CD8 T cells, as well as diminishes insulitis and diabetes onset in NOD mice [51]. Daily administration of a specific TLR7 ligand, 1V136, reduces autoimmune disease and modulates DC function [28]. In addition, treatment with 1Z1, an innate immune modulator generated by conjugating a TLR7 ligand to six units of polyethylene glycol (PEG), effectively prevented the clinical onset of hyperglycemia and reduced islet inflammation in NOD mice [52].

The involvement of TLR9 in T1D has been demonstrated in a rat model (diabetes-resistant BioBreeding or BBDR), which developed the disease following virus infection. In this study, disease progression was dependent on TLR9 signaling, leading to the activation of splenic B cells and bone marrow derived DCs [53]. A recent study investigating DCs subpopulations and their responses to TLRs stimulation in T1D patients, and their relatives showed increased TLR9-mediated interferon-alpha production in the first-degree relatives of T1D patients [27].

3. Contribution of TLRs to T1D complications

Diabetes leads to both microvascular and macrovascular complications. Many studies have shown increased levels of inflammatory biomarkers that could predispose to vascular complications. It is undeniable that TLRs are emerging as major factors in many diseases conditions owing to the activation of signaling pathways leading to the expression of inflammatory mediators and induction of immune responses.

Importantly, members of the TLR family play critical roles in the inflammatory components of vascular pathologies, including atherosclerosis [54-55], a condition characterized by inflammation of the vessel wall of the arterial tree. Atherosclerosis is an important vascular complication and the major cause of morbidity and mortality in diabetic patients [56]. Also, diabetes itself is a risk factor for atherosclerosis. Despite the fact that type 1 diabetics are at lower risk for atherosclerotic cardiovascular disease than type 2 diabetics because of the younger age of the former group, the relative risk is 10 times higher in type 1 diabetics than in nondiabetics of similar age [57]. Moreover, T1D has been linked with increased intima media thickness and impaired endothelial function (6), which affects vascular homeostasis leading to complications in diabetes. Lastly, hyperglycemia is a hallmark of diabetes and the role of glucose in the pathogenesis of atherosclerosis has been intensely discussed [58].

Devaraj et al. [30] reported on the role of TLR2 in the proinflammatory state in diabetes and incipient diabetic nephropathy. In TLR2 knockout streptozotocin (STZ)-induced diabetic animals, these authors observed a significant reduction in the NF-κB activity in peritoneal macrophages as well as in the release of various pro-inflammatory cytokines such as IL-6 and IL-8 compared to wild-type diabetic mice. Moreover, TLR2 KO STZ mice showed a significant decreased in albuminuria compared to WT-STZ, as well as increase in podocyte (epithelial cell in the kidneys) number, decrease in podocyte effacement, and a decrease in macrophages in the kidney. This study clearly implicates the TLR pathway in the genesis of a vascular complication in diabetes and demonstrates greater TLR activity in T1D.

Reactive oxygen species (ROS) formed in the vascular wall target a wide range of signaling molecules in both endothelium and vascular smooth muscle and contribute to vascular damage. Vascular dysfunction and remodeling through oxidative damage involves increased production and/or decreased degradation of ROS. One of the main enzymes implicated in vascular ROS generation is NADPH oxidase, although the mechanism behind induction of vascular NADPH oxidase activation in diabetes is less clear [59]. Recently, the role of TLRs in increased ROS levels in diabetes has been investigated [60-61]. It has been shown that the KO of the P47^{phox} subunit of NADPH oxidase prevents diet-induced obesity via upregulation of both TLR2 and TLR4 [61]. A study addressing diabetic retinopathy using human retinal endothelial treated with high glucose showed that hyperglycemia induces TLR2 and TLR4 activation and downstream TLR signaling mediates augmented inflammation possibly via ROS [62], suggesting a mechanism by which TLRs could contribute to vascular damage in diabetes. However, the precise ligands involved in the activation of TLRs by hyperglycemia are still under investigation, and certainly this information will provide new insight for a role of TLRs in diabetes-associated vascular complications.

4. Endogenous ligands (DAMPS) for TLRs in the mechanism of T1D

A large number of endogenous molecules may be potent activators of the innate immune system via TLRs leading to the release of proinflammatory cytokines from monocytes/macrophages. Unfortunately, there are limited data on the levels of endogenous ligands of TLR2 and TLR4 in T1D; however, a significant elevation of some ligands for TLR2 and TLR4 in T2D has been recently found. Overall, S100, fibrinogen, hyaluronan, oxidized LDL, and advanced glycation end products (AGE) showed increased levels in diabetic conditions and may work as DAMPS for TLRs [63]. However, high-mobility group box-1 protein (HMGB1), heat shock proteins (HSPs), and growth arrest-specific 6 protein (GAS6) are the ligands for TLRs specifically associated with T1D have been highlighted in the current literature.

4.1. HMGB1

HMGB1 was initially identified nearly 30 years ago as a chromatin associated protein that is important for transcriptional regulation. HMGB1 helps organize DNA and facilitates the binding of several regulatory protein complexes to DNA [64]. In addition to its role in transcriptional regulation, HMGB1 has been shown to activate proinflammatory responses following its release by necrotic or injured cells into the extracellular environment [65]. This protein may also be actively secreted by monocytes/macrophages. HMGB1 is implicated in the pathogenesis of a number of diseases associated with inflammation and tissue injury [66], and recently, many studies have suggested that HMGB1 acts as an inflammatory trigger in autoimmune diseases working as a DAMP [67]. Although the receptor for advanced glycation end products (RAGE) was the first HMGB1 receptor to be identified, this interaction alone could not justify all of the observed effects of HMGB1 [68]. Many relevant reports have shown that HMGB1 binds not only to RAGE, but also to TLRs [69]. The group of receptors that respond to HMGB1 is still expanding and includes cell membrane expressed TLR4 and TLR2 and endosomal TLR3, TLR7, and TLR9 [70].

To date, the main TLRs implicated in HMGB1 signaling are TLR2 and TLR4, although it is unknown if these receptors are acting independently or together. HMGB1 function is altered in diabetes, and the signaling systems triggered by this protein are not completely understood. The levels of TLRs and HMGB1 have been shown to be increased in patients with T1D [71], and HMGB1 is highly expressed in the cytoplasm of the islets in diabetic mice compared with nondiabetic controls. Furthermore, HMGB1 has been observed to increase in the cytoplasm of the islets during the progression of diabetes [72], and the augmented expression of this protein was observed in the retinas of diabetic patients with retinopathy [73].

HMGB1 polypeptide by itself has a weak proinflammatory activity, but it acquires proinflammatory activity through binding to proinflammatory mediators [74]. It is of interest to note that high glucose concentrations upregulate HMGB1, a ligand to TLR2 and TLR4 known to produce inflammation through NF-κB activation in human endothelial cells [69]. A recent study showed that while infusion of small amounts of glucose results in oxidative and inflammatory stress in patients with T1D, insulin infusion exerts an anti-inflammatory effect by suppression of TLRs and HMGB1 in mononuclear cells of T1D patients [75]. Moreover, it has been suggested that the activation of TLR4 and RAGE by HMGB1 mediates injury and inflammation by the activation of NF-κB in response to hyperglycemia [68]. A study using NOD mice to address the significance of HMGB1 in the natural history of diabetes showed that HMGB1 interacts with TLR4 in isolated islets. By examining the effects of anti-TLR4 antibodies on HMGB1 cell surfacing binding, the authors suggested that TLR4 is the main receptor for HMGB1 on beta-cells and that HMGB1 may signal through TLR4 to selectively impair beta-cells during the progression of T1D [72]. Overall, a considerable body of evidence suggests that a complex set of mechanisms involving HMGB1, RAGE, and TLRs play a significant role in the development of chronic inflammation in diabetes [68].

On the other hand, many studies have shown that HMGB1 has angiogenic properties in promoting endothelial cell sprouting and migration under hypoxic and necrotic conditions [76-77]. There are data suggesting that release of HMGB1 in wounds initiates TLR4-dependent responses that contribute to neovascularization [78]. In addition, research on the transcriptional profiles of angiogenic endothelial cells has revealed HMGB1 as a promising angiogenic factor [79]. Conversely, a potential role for HMGB1 in atherosclerosis [80] is possible, shown by increased HMGB1 expression in atherosclerotic lesions compared with normal arteries. Under some circumstances, HMGB1 may act as a double-edged sword, but it appears that HMGB1 as a ligand for TLRs in T1D plays a detrimental action. Despite these apparent conflicting results, HMGB1 has a central role in mediating local and systemic responses to several stimuli, is involved in TLRs pathways, and may have therapeutic relevance in T1D.

4.2. HSPs

Heat shock proteins (HSPs) were originally identified as a set of proteins that are upregulated by increases in temperature [81]. These proteins were named for their apparent molecular weight, for example, HSP70 and HSP60, and have been shown to be among the most highly conserved proteins in the cell. Some HSPs, like HSP60s, are already abundant proteins that are further upregulated during stressful conditions. Other HSPs, like HSP70, have homologues that are constitutively highly expressed (sometimes referred to as HSC70s) and other homologues that are stress inducible. Most HSPs function as molecular chaperones that assist in the folding of newly synthesized, misfolded, or damaged proteins. Their requirement in protein folding helps to explain the important role of HSPs in both stress and nonstress conditions and the high degree of HSP conservation.

In addition to their primary role in intracellular protein folding, HSPs have been co-opted in a variety of other pathways. HSPs play an important role in cellular pathways involving cellular growth, division, and apoptosis. HSPs have also been implicated in various aspects of immune system modulation [82]. For example, HSPs have been shown to be involved in antigen presentation through their ability to bind and traffic proteins and peptides.

While their primary function is inside the cell, during stress, HSPs can be expressed on cell surfaces or secreted. One of their extracellular functions is the cross presentation of various antigens that they can bind. In addition, extracellular and purified HSP70 and HSP60 have been shown to bind to TLR2 and TLR4, which results in NF-κB activation in a MyD88 and CD14-dependent manner [83]. HSPs can activate immune cells, including B cells, NK cells,

DCs, macrophages, and T cells. However, these results have been somewhat controversial as some HSP preparations have been shown to be contaminated with bacterial molecules, including LPS. Nevertheless, the abundance of HSPs, their high level of conservation, and their roles in cellular stress and inflammation may all help to explain why HSPs have been classified as important components of DAMP signals.

HSP60 and HSP70 have been implicated as key players in T1D. Both mouse models of T1D (NOD mice) and human patients have T cells that recognize and are activated by HSP60 and HSP70 [84-86]. These activated T cells then go to the pancreatic islets and recognize self HSP60 as an autoantigen. Extracellular HSP70 levels are positively correlated with insulin resistance *in vivo* and can cause β-cell dysfunction and death *in vitro* [87]. In mouse models, exogenous HSP60 and immunogenic peptides from HSP60 have been shown to alter the effects of T cells and prevent further β-cell destruction [88]. One peptide, in particular, DiaPep277, has shown promise in phase II clinical trials [89-90]. Phase III clinical trials using this peptide have been completed, but problems with the data analysis have surfaced and a new analysis of the clinical data is currently underway and expected to be completed soon [91-92]. HSP60 and HSP70 have also been implicated in complications of T1D, including atherosclerosis, indicating that they may have multiple roles in T1D [93-95].

4.3. GAS6

Growth arrest-specific 6 (GAS6) protein is another endogenous ligand of TLR2 and TLR4 that has been studied in experimental models of diabetic nephropathy [96], which is the most common cause of end-stage renal diseases, affecting 30% of T1D patients [97]. GAS6 and its receptor Axl play a key role in the development of glomerular hypertrophy, a hallmark of the early phase of nephropathy. In diabetic rats, it has been demonstrated that GAS6/Axl mediates glomerular hypertrophy during diabetes [96]. However, there is a paucity of information about the association of GAS6 and TLRs, and the involvement of GAS6 as a ligand for TLRs in T1D is unknown. Recently, analyzing the levels of ligands of TLR2 and TLR4 in mononuclear cells isolated from blood samples collected in patients with T1D, Deveraj and coworkers showed increased levels of HSP60 and HMGB1, but no significant difference in the levels of GAS6 between T1D diabetic group and their matched controls [71]. Therefore, further studies are necessary to clarify if there is a link between GAS6 and TLRs in the pathogenesis of T1D.

5. Targeting TLRs to manage T1D

Studies into the mechanisms behind disease progression have tended focus on identifying the important cell types and pathways involved in T1D. Definitely, TLR pathways are involved in T1D, making these receptors a tempting immune-based therapeutic intervention to handle T1D. TLR2 and TLR4 have a potential role in mediating inflammation and consequently, the complications associated with diabetes, mainly vascular damage, making them attractive targets. The deficiency of TLR4 as well as TLR2 is associated with reduced atherosclerosis and inflammatory state in diabetic mice [30, 98]. Treatment with a TLR4 antagonist was shown to inhibit vascular inflammation and atherogenesis in STZ-induced ApoE$^{-/-}$ diabetic mice, as well as lower serum cholesterol and triglyceride levels in nondiabetic ApoE$^{-/-}$ mice [99]. It has been shown that TLR9$^{-/-}$ NOD mice present a delay in the onset of diabetes with decreased IFN-α production and decreased diabetogenic CD8 T cells in pancreatic lymph nodes. Moreover, the addition of a TLR9 antagonist oligodeoxynucleotide or chloroquine inhibited bone-marrow-derived DCs activation and CD8 T cells priming in response to CpG, an agonist of TLR9 [100].

Conversely, TLR agonists have been successfully used in NOD mice to delay T1D by inducing tolerogenic responses [39, 101]. The TLR2 agonist Pam3CSK4, when administered chronically in NOD mice, inhibits the development of T1D. Also, diabetogenic T cell priming of DCs was attenuated by chronic treatment with Pam3CSK4, suggesting DC tolerance [20]. Furthermore, the combination of TLR2 tolerization and inhibition of dipeptydil peptidase 4 (DPP4), which has been demonstrated to ameliorate STZ-induced diabetes by increasing beta-cell mass [102], can reverse early-onset diabetes in NOD mice [101].

Briefly, two contradictory possibilities have been considered regarding TLRs as a target to manage T1D. One is based on the belief that TLRs mediate T1D onset and its complications. Therefore, targeting these receptors using antibody treatment, pharmacological antagonist, or genetic approaches could minimize diabetes complications and decrease inflammation. The second possibility is based on the strategy of inhibiting T1D by tolerance mechanisms. There are scientific reports for both possibilities, making these receptors an attractive future option for treatment of T1D. However, the exact role of TLRs in the pathogenesis of T1D is not completely understood and the initial event of T1D is not revealed. Therefore, therapeutic approaches for T1D using TLR targeting remain a mere theoretical alternative.

6. Conclusion

The idea that the upregulation of TLR pathways, under some circumstances, leads to the induction of proinflammatory responses, and islet destruction is consistent with emerging data in animal models of T1D. In addition, a large body of evidence suggests increased TLR activity in diabetic patients, and these receptors have been suggested to be involved in the pathogenesis of diabetic vasculopathies. Therefore, therapeutic strategies to prevent TLR-mediated inflammation in T1D via modulation of either receptors or their DAMPs ligands can be a welcome addition to the available approaches to deal with T1D and diabetic vascular complications. However, targeting TLRs themselves using approaches such as antagonists could pose the risk of compromising host immunity. In addition, while some antigen-based immunotherapies targeting TLR ligands have proven to be protective against T1D development in animal models, these protocols might not be successfully adaptable to human diabetic patients at the time of diagnosis due to the nature of pathogenic and tolerogenic antigen selection in animal models and human individuals [103].

In fact, there exist number crucial questions regarding TLRs and T1D mechanisms that remain to be addressed. One of the major questions is do TLR pathways promote the initiation or effector phase of diabetes, or both? A more complete understanding of how the innate immune system via TLRs can modulate autoimmune responses to beta-cell antigens, as well as the mechanisms by which these receptors are contributing to triggering and tuning T1D is crucial, not only because this information can lead to clear elucidation of the role of the innate immune system in TD1 but also because it may clarify whether TLRs can be used as an innovative clinical approach to manage or prevent this disease.

Acknowledgements

Doctor Nunes and Dr. Webb are supported by American Heart Association (Scientific Development Grant, SDG 12080023 and Grant-in-Aid, respectively).

Author details

Kenia Pedrosa Nunes[1*], Eric Guisbert[1], Theodora Szasz[2] and Clinton Webb[2]

*Address all correspondence to: keniapedrosa@gmail.com

1 Department of Biological Sciences, Florida Institute of Technology, Melbourne, FL, USA

2 Department of Physiology, Georgia Regents University, Augusta, GA, USA

References

[1] Janeway, C.A., Jr. and R. Medzhitov, *Innate immune recognition*. Annu Rev Immunol, 2002. 20: p. 197-216.

[2] Meylan, E., J. Tschopp, and M. Karin, *Intracellular pattern recognition receptors in the host response*. Nature, 2006. 442(7098): p. 39-44.

[3] O'Neill, L.A., D. Golenbock, and A.G. Bowie, *The history of Toll-like receptors - redefining innate immunity*. Nat Rev Immunol, 2013. 13(6): p. 453-60.

[4] Lee, C.C., A.M. Avalos, and H.L. Ploegh, *Accessory molecules for Toll-like receptors and their function*. Nat Rev Immunol, 2012. 12(3): p. 168-79.

[5] Assmann, T.S., et al., *Toll-like receptor 3 (TLR3) and the development of type 1 diabetes mellitus*. Arch Endocrinol Metab, 2015. 59(1): p. 4-12.

[6] Devaraj, S., et al., *Increased toll-like receptor (TLR) 2 and TLR4 expression in monocytes from patients with type 1 diabetes: further evidence of a proinflammatory state*. J Clin Endocrinol Metab, 2008. 93(2): p. 578-83.

[7] Schranz, D.B. and A. Lernmark, *Immunology in diabetes: an update.* Diabetes Metab Rev, 1998. 14(1): p. 3-29.

[8] Lien, E. and D. Zipris, *The role of Toll-like receptor pathways in the mechanism of type 1 diabetes.* Curr Mol Med, 2009. 9(1): p. 52-68.

[9] Zipris, D., *Epidemiology of type 1 diabetes and what animal models teach us about the role of viruses in disease mechanisms.* Clin Immunol, 2009. 131(1): p. 11-23.

[10] Todd, J.A., J.I. Bell, and H.O. McDevitt, *HLA-DQ beta gene contributes to susceptibility and resistance to insulin-dependent diabetes mellitus.* Nature, 1987. 329(6140): p. 599-604.

[11] Todd, J.A., et al., *Genetic analysis of autoimmune type 1 diabetes mellitus in mice.* Nature, 1991. 351(6327): p. 542-7.

[12] Rewers, M. and P. Zimmet, *The rising tide of childhood type 1 diabetes--what is the elusive environmental trigger?* Lancet, 2004. 364(9446): p. 1645-7.

[13] Eizirik, D.L. and T. Mandrup-Poulsen, *A choice of death--the signal-transduction of immune-mediated beta-cell apoptosis.* Diabetologia, 2001. 44(12): p. 2115-33.

[14] Komai-Koma, M., et al., *TLR2 is expressed on activated T cells as a costimulatory receptor.* Proc Natl Acad Sci U S A, 2004. 101(9): p. 3029-34.

[15] Jin, B., et al., *The effects of TLR activation on T-cell development and differentiation.* Clin Dev Immunol, 2012. 2012: p. 836485.

[16] Hua, Z. and B. Hou, *TLR signaling in B-cell development and activation.* Cell Mol Immunol, 2013. 10(2): p. 103-6.

[17] Santoni, M., et al., *Toll like receptors and pancreatic diseases: From a pathogenetic mechanism to a therapeutic target.* Cancer Treat Rev, 2015. 41(7): p. 569-76.

[18] Diana, J., et al., *Innate immunity in type 1 diabetes.* Discov Med, 2011. 11(61): p. 513-20.

[19] Lee, M.S., *Role of innate immunity in the pathogenesis of type 1 and type 2 diabetes.* J Korean Med Sci, 2014. 29(8): p. 1038-41.

[20] Lee, M.S., *Treatment of autoimmune diabetes by inhibiting the initial event.* Immune Netw, 2013. 13(5): p. 194-8.

[21] Steinman, R.M., D. Hawiger, and M.C. Nussenzweig, *Tolerogenic dendritic cells.* Annu Rev Immunol, 2003. 21: p. 685-711.

[22] Hammond, T., et al., *Toll-like receptor (TLR) expression on CD4+ and CD8+ T-cells in patients chronically infected with hepatitis C virus.* Cell Immunol, 2010. 264(2): p. 150-5.

[23] Schram, M.T., et al., *Markers of inflammation are cross-sectionally associated with microvascular complications and cardiovascular disease in type 1 diabetes--the EURODIAB Prospective Complications Study.* Diabetologia, 2005. 48(2): p. 370-8.

[24] Devaraj, S., et al., *Evidence of increased inflammation and microcirculatory abnormalities in patients with type 1 diabetes and their role in microvascular complications.* Diabetes, 2007. 56(11): p. 2790-6.

[25] Devaraj, S., et al., *Demonstration of increased toll-like receptor 2 and toll-like receptor 4 expression in monocytes of type 1 diabetes mellitus patients with microvascular complications.* Metabolism, 2011. 60(2): p. 256-9.

[26] Li, H. and B. Sun, *Toll-like receptor 4 in atherosclerosis.* J Cell Mol Med, 2007. 11(1): p. 88-95.

[27] Kayserova, J., et al., *Decreased dendritic cell numbers but increased TLR9-mediated interferon-alpha production in first degree relatives of type 1 diabetes patients.* Clin Immunol, 2014. 153(1): p. 49-55.

[28] Hayashi, T., et al., *Treatment of autoimmune inflammation by a TLR7 ligand regulating the innate immune system.* PLoS One, 2012. 7(9): p. e45860.

[29] Karumuthil-Melethil, S., et al., *TLR2- and Dectin 1-associated innate immune response modulates T-cell response to pancreatic beta-cell antigen and prevents type 1 diabetes.* Diabetes, 2015. 64(4): p. 1341-57.

[30] Devaraj, S., et al., *Knockout of toll-like receptor-2 attenuates both the proinflammatory state of diabetes and incipient diabetic nephropathy.* Arterioscler Thromb Vasc Biol, 2011. 31(8): p. 1796-804.

[31] Sakata, Y., et al., *Toll-like receptor 2 modulates left ventricular function following ischemia-reperfusion injury.* Am J Physiol Heart Circ Physiol, 2007. 292(1): p. H503-9.

[32] Devaraj, S. and I. Jialal, *Increased secretion of IP-10 from monocytes under hyperglycemia is via the TLR2 and TLR4 pathway.* Cytokine, 2009. 47(1): p. 6-10.

[33] Kim, D.H., et al., *Inhibition of autoimmune diabetes by TLR2 tolerance.* J Immunol, 2011. 187(10): p. 5211-20.

[34] Dasu, M.R., et al., *TLR2 expression and signaling-dependent inflammation impair wound healing in diabetic mice.* Lab Invest, 2010. 90(11): p. 1628-36.

[35] Mudaliar, H., et al., *The role of TLR2 and 4-mediated inflammatory pathways in endothelial cells exposed to high glucose.* PLoS One, 2014. 9(10): p. e108844.

[36] Shigihara, T., et al., *Significance of serum CXCL10/IP-10 level in type 1 diabetes.* J Autoimmun, 2006. 26(1): p. 66-71.

[37] Caramalho, I., et al., *Regulatory T cells selectively express toll-like receptors and are activated by lipopolysaccharide.* J Exp Med, 2003. 197(4): p. 403-11.

[38] Liu, H., et al., *Toll-like receptor 2 signaling modulates the functions of CD4+ CD25+ regulatory T cells.* Proc Natl Acad Sci U S A, 2006. 103(18): p. 7048-53.

[39] Filippi, C.M., et al., *TLR2 signaling improves immunoregulation to prevent type 1 diabetes.* Eur J Immunol, 2011. 41(5): p. 1399-409.

[40] Wen, L., et al., *Innate immunity and intestinal microbiota in the development of Type 1 diabetes.* Nature, 2008. 455(7216): p. 1109-13.

[41] Kachapati, K., et al., *The non-obese diabetic (NOD) mouse as a model of human type 1 diabetes.* Methods Mol Biol, 2012. 933: p. 3-16.

[42] Kim, H.S., et al., *Toll-like receptor 2 senses beta-cell death and contributes to the initiation of autoimmune diabetes.* Immunity, 2007. 27(2): p. 321-33.

[43] Gulden, E., et al., *Toll-like receptor 4 deficiency accelerates the development of insulin-deficient diabetes in non-obese diabetic mice.* PLoS One, 2013. 8(9): p. e75385.

[44] Dong, B., et al., *TLR4 regulates cardiac lipid accumulation and diabetic heart disease in the nonobese diabetic mouse model of type 1 diabetes.* Am J Physiol Heart Circ Physiol, 2012. 303(6): p. H732-42.

[45] Bednar, K.J. and W.M. Ridgway, *Targeting innate immunity for treatment of type 1 diabetes.* Immunotherapy, 2014. 6(12): p. 1239-42.

[46] Bednar, K.J., et al., *Reversal of New-Onset Type 1 Diabetes with an agonistic TLR4/MD-2 Monoclonal Antibody.* Diabetes, 2015.

[47] Vallois, D., et al., *The type 1 diabetes locus Idd6 controls TLR1 expression.* J Immunol, 2007. 179(6): p. 3896-903.

[48] Assmann, T.S., et al., *Polymorphisms in the TLR3 gene are associated with risk for type 1 diabetes mellitus.* Eur J Endocrinol, 2014. 170(4): p. 519-27.

[49] Pirie, F.J., et al., *Toll-like receptor 3 gene polymorphisms in South African Blacks with type 1 diabetes.* Tissue Antigens, 2005. 66(2): p. 125-30.

[50] Coppieters, K.T., T. Boettler, and M. von Herrath, *Virus infections in type 1 diabetes.* Cold Spring Harb Perspect Med, 2012. 2(1): p. a007682.

[51] Lee, A.S., et al., *Toll-like receptor 7 stimulation promotes autoimmune diabetes in the NOD mouse.* Diabetologia, 2011. 54(6): p. 1407-16.

[52] Hayashi, T., et al., *Induction of Tolerogenic Dendritic Cells by a PEGylated TLR7 Ligand for Treatment of Type 1 Diabetes.* PLoS One, 2015. 10(6): p. e0129867.

[53] Zipris, D., et al., *TLR9-signaling pathways are involved in Kilham rat virus-induced autoimmune diabetes in the biobreeding diabetes-resistant rat.* J Immunol, 2007. 178(2): p. 693-701.

[54] Edfeldt, K., et al., *Expression of toll-like receptors in human atherosclerotic lesions: a possible pathway for plaque activation.* Circulation, 2002. 105(10): p. 1158-61.

[55] Curtiss, L.K. and P.S. Tobias, *Emerging role of Toll-like receptors in atherosclerosis.* J Lipid Res, 2009. 50 Suppl: p. S340-5.

[56] Swerdlow, A.J. and M.E. Jones, *Mortality during 25 years of follow-up of a cohort with diabetes.* Int J Epidemiol, 1996. 25(6): p. 1250-61.

[57] Soedamah-Muthu, S.S., et al., *High risk of cardiovascular disease in patients with type 1 diabetes in the U.K.: a cohort study using the general practice research database.* Diabetes Care, 2006. 29(4): p. 798-804.

[58] Chait, A. and K.E. Bornfeldt, *Diabetes and atherosclerosis: is there a role for hyperglycemia?* J Lipid Res, 2009. 50 Suppl: p. S335-9.

[59] Yung, L.M., et al., *Reactive oxygen species in vascular wall.* Cardiovasc Hematol Disord Drug Targets, 2006. 6(1): p. 1-19.

[60] Asehnoune, K., et al., *Involvement of reactive oxygen species in Toll-like receptor 4-dependent activation of NF-kappa B.* J Immunol, 2004. 172(4): p. 2522-9.

[61] Chen, J.X. and A. Stinnett, *Critical role of the NADPH oxidase subunit p47phox on vascular TLR expression and neointimal lesion formation in high-fat diet-induced obesity.* Lab Invest, 2008. 88(12): p. 1316-28.

[62] Rajamani, U. and I. Jialal, *Hyperglycemia induces Toll-like receptor-2 and -4 expression and activity in human microvascular retinal endothelial cells: implications for diabetic retinopathy.* J Diabetes Res, 2014. 2014: p. 790902.

[63] Shin, J.J., et al., *Damage-associated molecular patterns and their pathological relevance in diabetes mellitus.* Ageing Res Rev, 2015.

[64] Lotze, M.T. and K.J. Tracey, *High-mobility group box 1 protein (HMGB1): nuclear weapon in the immune arsenal.* Nat Rev Immunol, 2005. 5(4): p. 331-42.

[65] Wang, H., H. Yang, and K.J. Tracey, *Extracellular role of HMGB1 in inflammation and sepsis.* J Intern Med, 2004. 255(3): p. 320-31.

[66] Tang, D., et al., *High-mobility group box 1, oxidative stress, and disease.* Antioxid Redox Signal, 2011. 14(7): p. 1315-35.

[67] Lotze, M.T., A. Deisseroth, and A. Rubartelli, *Damage associated molecular pattern molecules.* Clin Immunol, 2007. 124(1): p. 1-4.

[68] Nogueira-Machado, J.A., et al., *HMGB1, TLR and RAGE: a functional tripod that leads to diabetic inflammation.* Expert Opin Ther Targets, 2011. 15(8): p. 1023-35.

[69] Park, J.S., et al., *High mobility group box 1 protein interacts with multiple Toll-like receptors.* Am J Physiol Cell Physiol, 2006. 290(3): p. C917-24.

[70] Branco-Madeira, F. and B.N. Lambrecht, *High mobility group box-1 recognition: the beginning of a RAGEless era?* EMBO Mol Med, 2010. 2(6): p. 193-5.

[71]   Devaraj, S., et al., *Increased levels of ligands of Toll-like receptors 2 and 4 in type 1 diabetes.* Diabetologia, 2009. 52(8): p. 1665-8.

[72]   Li, M., et al., *Toll-like receptor 4 on islet beta cells senses expression changes in high-mobility group box 1 and contributes to the initiation of type 1 diabetes.* Exp Mol Med, 2012. 44(4): p. 260-7.

[73]   Dasu, M.R., et al., *Increased toll-like receptor (TLR) activation and TLR ligands in recently diagnosed type 2 diabetic subjects.* Diabetes Care, 2010. 33(4): p. 861-8.

[74]   Li, J., et al., *Recombinant HMGB1 with cytokine-stimulating activity.* J Immunol Methods, 2004. 289(1-2): p. 211-23.

[75]   Dandona, P., et al., *Insulin infusion suppresses while glucose infusion induces Toll-like receptors and high-mobility group-B1 protein expression in mononuclear cells of type 1 diabetes patients.* Am J Physiol Endocrinol Metab, 2013. 304(8): p. E810-8.

[76]   Schlueter, C., et al., *Angiogenetic signaling through hypoxia: HMGB1: an angiogenetic switch molecule.* Am J Pathol, 2005. 166(4): p. 1259-63.

[77]   Biscetti, F., et al., *High-mobility group box-1 protein promotes angiogenesis after peripheral ischemia in diabetic mice through a VEGF-dependent mechanism.* Diabetes, 2010. 59(6): p. 1496-505.

[78]   Lin, Q., et al., *High-mobility group box-1 mediates toll-like receptor 4-dependent angiogenesis.* Arterioscler Thromb Vasc Biol, 2011. 31(5): p. 1024-32.

[79]   van Beijnum, J.R., et al., *Gene expression of tumor angiogenesis dissected: specific targeting of colon cancer angiogenic vasculature.* Blood, 2006. 108(7): p. 2339-48.

[80]   Porto, A., et al., *Smooth muscle cells in human atherosclerotic plaques secrete and proliferate in response to high mobility group box 1 protein.* FASEB J, 2006. 20(14): p. 2565-6.

[81]   Guisbert, E., et al., *Identification of a tissue-selective heat shock response regulatory network.* PLoS Genet, 2013. 9(4): p. e1003466.

[82]   Tsan, M.F. and B. Gao, *Heat shock proteins and immune system.* J Leukoc Biol, 2009. 85(6): p. 905-10.

[83]   Asea, A., *Heat shock proteins and toll-like receptors.* Handb Exp Pharmacol, 2008(183): p. 111-27.

[84]   Abulafia-Lapid, R., et al., *T cells and autoantibodies to human HSP70 in type 1 diabetes in children.* J Autoimmun, 2003. 20(4): p. 313-21.

[85]   Abulafia-Lapid, R., et al., *T cell proliferative responses of type 1 diabetes patients and healthy individuals to human hsp60 and its peptides.* J Autoimmun, 1999. 12(2): p. 121-9.

[86]   Birk, O.S., et al., *NOD mouse diabetes: the ubiquitous mouse hsp60 is a beta-cell target antigen of autoimmune T cells.* J Autoimmun, 1996. 9(2): p. 159-66.

[87] Krause, M., et al., *Elevated levels of extracellular heat-shock protein 72 (eHSP72) are posi-tively correlated with insulin resistance in vivo and cause pancreatic beta-cell dysfunction and death in vitro.* Clin Sci (Lond), 2014. 126(10): p. 739-52.

[88] Bockova, J., D. Elias, and I.R. Cohen, *Treatment of NOD diabetes with a novel peptide of the hsp60 molecule induces Th2-type antibodies.* J Autoimmun, 1997. 10(4): p. 323-9.

[89] Raz, I., et al., *Treatment of new-onset type 1 diabetes with peptide DiaPep277 is safe and associated with preserved beta-cell function: extension of a randomized, double-blind, phase II trial.* Diabetes Metab Res Rev, 2007. 23(4): p. 292-8.

[90] Raz, I., et al., *Beta-cell function in new-onset type 1 diabetes and immunomodulation with a heat-shock protein peptide (DiaPep277): a randomised, double-blind, phase II trial.* Lancet, 2001. 358(9295): p. 1749-53.

[91] *Treatment of recent-onset type 1 diabetic patients with DiaPep277: results of a double-blind, placebo-controlled, randomized phase 3 trial. Diabetes Care 2014;37:1392-1400. DOI: 10.2337/dc13-1391.* Diabetes Care, 2015. 38(1): p. 178.

[92] Raz, I., et al., *Treatment of recent-onset type 1 diabetic patients with DiaPep277: results of a double-blind, placebo-controlled, randomized phase 3 trial.* Diabetes Care, 2014. 37(5): p. 1392-400.

[93] Rajaiah, R. and K.D. Moudgil, *Heat-shock proteins can promote as well as regulate autoim-munity.* Autoimmun Rev, 2009. 8(5): p. 388-93.

[94] Noble, E.G. and G.X. Shen, *Impact of exercise and metabolic disorders on heat shock pro-teins and vascular inflammation.* Autoimmune Dis, 2012. 2012: p. 836519.

[95] Qu, B., et al., *The detection and role of heat shock protein 70 in various nondisease condi-tions and disease conditions: a literature review.* Cell Stress Chaperones, 2015.

[96] Nagai, K., et al., *Growth arrest-specific gene 6 is involved in glomerular hypertrophy in the early stage of diabetic nephropathy.* J Biol Chem, 2003. 278(20): p. 18229-34.

[97] Bojestig, M., et al., *Declining incidence of nephropathy in insulin-dependent diabetes melli-tus.* N Engl J Med, 1994. 330(1): p. 15-8.

[98] Devaraj, S., P. Tobias, and I. Jialal, *Knockout of toll-like receptor-4 attenuates the pro-in-flammatory state of diabetes.* Cytokine, 2011. 55(3): p. 441-5.

[99] Lu, Z., et al., *TLR4 antagonist reduces early-stage atherosclerosis in diabetic apolipoprotein E-deficient mice.* J Endocrinol, 2013. 216(1): p. 61-71.

[100] Zhang, Y., et al., *TLR9 blockade inhibits activation of diabetogenic CD8+ T cells and delays autoimmune diabetes.* J Immunol, 2010. 184(10): p. 5645-53.

[101] Kim, D.H., et al., *Treatment of autoimmune diabetes in NOD mice by Toll-like receptor 2 tolerance in conjunction with dipeptidyl peptidase 4 inhibition.* Diabetologia, 2012. 55(12): p. 3308-17.

[102] Cho, J.M., et al., *A novel dipeptidyl peptidase IV inhibitor DA-1229 ameliorates streptozoto-cin-induced diabetes by increasing beta-cell replication and neogenesis*. Diabetes Res Clin Pract, 2011. 91(1): p. 72-9.

[103] Serreze, D.V. and Y.G. Chen, *Of mice and men: use of animal models to identify possible interventions for the prevention of autoimmune type 1 diabetes in humans*. Trends Immunol, 2005. 26(11): p. 603-7.

Permissions

The contributors of this book come from diverse backgrounds, making this book a truly international effort. This book will bring forth new frontiers with its revolutionizing research information and detailed analysis of the nascent developments around the world.

We would like to thank all the contributing authors for lending their expertise to make the book truly unique. They have played a crucial role in the development of this book. Without their invaluable contributions this book wouldn't have been possible. They have made vital efforts to compile up to date information on the varied aspects of this subject to make this book a valuable addition to the collection of many professionals and students.

This book was conceptualized with the vision of imparting up-to-date information and advanced data in this field. To ensure the same, a matchless editorial board was set up. Every individual on the board went through rigorous rounds of assessment to prove their worth. After which they invested a large part of their time researching and compiling the most relevant data for our readers.

The editorial board has been involved in producing this book since its inception. They have spent rigorous hours researching and exploring the diverse topics which have resulted in the successful publishing of this book. They have passed on their knowledge of decades through this book. To expedite this challenging task, the publisher supported the team at every step. A small team of assistant editors was also appointed to further simplify the editing procedure and attain best results for the readers.

Apart from the editorial board, the designing team has also invested a significant amount of their time in understanding the subject and creating the most relevant covers. They scrutinized every image to scout for the most suitable representation of the subject and create an appropriate cover for the book.

The publishing team has been an ardent support to the editorial, designing and production team. Their endless efforts to recruit the best for this project, has resulted in the accomplishment of this book. They are a veteran in the field of academics and their pool of knowledge is as vast as their experience in printing. Their expertise and guidance has proved useful at every step. Their uncompromising quality standards have made this book an exceptional effort. Their encouragement from time to time has been an inspiration for everyone.

The publisher and the editorial board hope that this book will prove to be a valuable piece of knowledge for researchers, students, practitioners and scholars across the globe.

List of Contributors

Efraim Berco, Daniel Rappoport, Ayala Pollack, Guy Kleinmann and Yoel Greenwald
Ophthalmology Department, Kaplan Medical Center, Rehovot, Israel
Hebrew University and Hadassah Medical School, Jerusalem, Israel

Kazuko Masuo
Baker IDI Heart & Diabetes Institute, Melbourne, Victoria, Australia

Michal Cohen and Smadar Shilo
Pediatric Diabetes Clinic and Pediatrics A Division, the Ruth Rappaport Children's Hospital, Rambam healthcare campus, Haifa, Israel

Nehama Zuckerman-Levin and Naim Shehadeh
Pediatric Diabetes Clinic and Pediatrics A Division, the Ruth Rappaport Children's Hospital, Rambam healthcare campus, Haifa, Israel
Rappaport Faculty of Medicine, Technion, Haifa, Israel

Fuad AlSaraj
Mediclinic Welcare Hospital, Dubai, UAE

Ippei Watari and Takashi Ono
Orthodontic Science, Department of Orofacial Development and Function, Division of Oral Health Science, Graduate School of Medical and Dental Science, Tokyo Medical and Dental University (TMDU), Tokyo, Japan

Mona Aly Abbassy
Department of Orthodontics, Faculty of Dentistry, King Abdulaziz University, Jeddah, Saudi Arabia
Alexandria University, Alexandria, Egypt

Katarzyna Anna Podyma-Inoue
Section of Biochemistry, Department of Bio-Matrix, Graduate School of Medical and Dental Science, Tokyo Medical and Dental University (TMDU), Tokyo, Japan

Kenia Pedrosa Nunes and Eric Guisbert
Department of Biological Sciences, Florida Institute of Technology, Melbourne, FL, USA

Theodora Szasz and Clinton Webb
Department of Physiology, Georgia Regents University, Augusta, GA, USA

Index

www.ingramcontent.com/pod-product-compliance
Lightning Source LLC
Chambersburg PA
CBHW062007190326
41458CB00009B/2998

* 9 7 8 1 6 3 2 4 2 6 4 9 9 *